The Pillars of Health

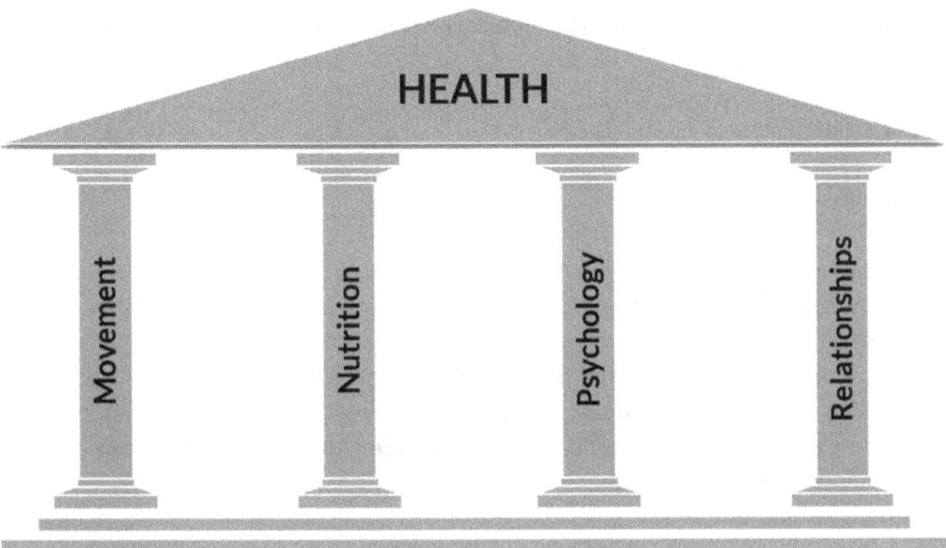

A Habit Based Approach to Cultivating Health and Reaching Your Potential

Corey Hobbs

Copyright Notice

All intellectual property from this text belongs to Corey Hobbs and CH Health & Fitness.

Legal Disclaimer: The advice given in the book is to be used at the reader's discretion. Corey J Hobbs, CH Health & Fitness, along with the publisher and contributors within this book disclaim any and all responsibility for any adverse effects, consequences, loss and/or damage as a result of the use/misuse of any information or suggestion within this book, as well as any presentations, consultations and clinics that are based upon its principles or their use. The information presented is based on my current knowledge of the topics. As I continue to grow, it is almost certain that these understandings will grow as well. If there is any confusion regarding any of these topics, reach out to a coach and allow them to help you through this process.

Thank you to my wife for always supporting me and all of my crazy ideas. Thank you to my son for teaching me how to love unconditionally and find joy in the little moments. I love you both more than I could ever describe.

Thank you to everyone who helped throughout this whole process from every mentor who helped me grow, to those first few people who went through the habits, and those that helped with suggestions and refinement. Without you all, this would not even exist.

Preface

Full Disclosure: Precision Nutrition has been doing habit-based nutrition coaching for a long time. They have been doing it for longer than I have. I would not be the coach that I am without the quality information the team at Precision Nutrition continues to put out. As a Strength and Conditioning Coach, I quickly realized that Nutrition can be a great performance enhancer when done correctly. That is why the Precision Nutrition Certification is the first one I sought. This book is by no means an attempt to dethrone what they have done. Instead, I hope it sheds light on the incredible methodologies and products that they have. For more information on Precision Nutrition head to https://www.precisionnutrition.com. They also have many additional resources that could be used to help you reach your goals. Many of these I share with my own clients frequently.

I wanted to bring this forward in a manner that resonates with my purpose, values, and goals to create a product that I can use in conjunction with my coaching to help people reach their goals. If you are familiar with Simon Sinek's work, you likely know the value of having a just cause to rally behind in conjunction with a strong why. My just cause is to eliminate chronic disease. My why is because despite spending more on healthcare as a nation, we are sicker than ever. Worse yet, the nutrition and health space are a confusing world of bad advice and false promises. I have spent an absurd amount of money on supplements, and I have tried all the tips and tricks. None of them work. I was a sucker, and I do not want the same thing to happen to others. It is my hope that this can help you avoid my mistakes by providing quality information in support of my just cause.

Not a lot of people understand what a Health or Nutrition Coach is or can do. I do not tell you what to eat or do because I want you to have the freedom to find what works best for your situation. That is where this book comes from. The desire to bring accessible information forward to anyone who may need it so that they can take control of their health and their life. Health is about so much more than the foods we eat and the exercise we partake in. I will dig into that more later, but for now, let us get into my story.

I am sure you are wondering something along the lines of "who the heck are you?", "what makes you qualified to do this?", or "why should I do these habits?" Those are all excellent questions. Allow me to introduce myself. My name is Corey Hobbs. I am a Strength and Conditioning Coach by trade. I am certified through the National Strength and Conditioning Association, Precision Nutrition, and a number of others that will not really make much sense to you unless you're in the field. You may notice that I do not place the alphabet soup of certifications or degrees behind my name like others in the field. There is nothing wrong with doing that. We work hard for those. However, I believe my story and journey is what allows me to be a good coach. My education certainly helps, but I would not be the person I am today if not for my own struggles (for a more in-depth introduction head to www.coreyhobbs.com).

I attended the United States Military Academy (USMA) where I received a degree in Kinesiology. I then served in the Army. Prior to my attendance at USMA, I went to Junior College in California. While attending Junior College and USMA, I played football. This is where my love of strength and conditioning first started. I was always much better in the weight room than I was on the field.

Throughout my adult life, my weight has fluctuated to as high as 280 lbs., and as low as 195 lbs. Throughout these fluctuations, the way in which I made it happen was not always the healthiest. We had to rush to lose weight after our final season of football to graduate. I actually had an extra year before graduation since I played in Junior College. So, I did not need to rush. However, my friends were doing it, and I felt that I had to struggle along with them. As the saying goes, that is just the way we do it around here. This is one of the most dangerous statements out there. It is the enemy of growth and improvement.

Thanks to having some of the best mentors around, and a drive to truly understand the body and the way it functions, I began the deep dive into nutrition and its implications for health and performance. It was not until I finally understood the importance of quality nutrition that I was able to be comfortable with who I am and the food I eat. I still struggle sometimes, and I am still an offensive lineman at heart (if you do not believe me, come visit when my wife bakes cookies. It will not take long to understand by how quickly I fall victim to the addictive properties of sugar). I have tried just about every diet, supplement, tip, and trick in the book. I battled with body image and a poor relationship with food. Yo-Yo dieting was a near constant in my life.

Now, as a Strength and Conditioning Coach, I get more questions about nutrition than strength. Nutrition is one of the easiest ways we can optimize our health and performance and reach our goals. However, thanks to the food industry, Instagram influencers with no real qualifications, advertising, and an overwhelming amount of information available today, the waters of nutrition are murky to say the least. Making nutrition easy in theory, but difficult in execution. We know we need to eat well to be healthy, but what does that even mean? With the information presented here, I hope to make nutrition easy in theory and in practice.

Thanks to the habits presented within this book, I have been able to get my own nutrition under control and help others do it too!

Contents

Contents 7

Section I: Introduction 10

   The Diet Problem 12

   How to Use this Book 24

Section II: Before the Food 34

   Habit 1: Make Time 36

   Habit 2: Slow Down 48

   Habit 3: Go to Sleep 59

   Habit 4: Build your Supporting Cast 70

Section III: The Food 86

   Habit 5: Water 89

   Habit 6: Protein 101

   Habit 7: Carbohydrates 114

   Habit 8: Fats 128

Section IV: Putting It All Together 146

   Habit 9: Pantry Shakedown 148

   Habit 10: Home Cooked Meals 161

   Habit 11: Move 171

   Habit 12: Live 184

Section V: The Next Level 188

   Supplements 190

   Avoiding Toxins 200

   Tackling Restaurants 207

Meditation 211

An Introduction to Functional Medicine 216

Closing Thoughts and Further Readings 223

Further Readings 226

Key Takeaways 229

All References 231

Section I: Introduction

This section serves as a tour guide so to speak. We will go over how you can use this book and the problem with the diet culture we currently face.

The Diet Problem

We have all been there: the number on the scale is higher than it has ever been, and the person in the mirror is not the same person from our peak physique. That is literally the reason I started my journey which resulted in the Pillars of Health. I saw a picture of myself from my wedding ceremony, and I knew that I was not healthy. I thought I was. I thought I had things figured out. I was strong, could pass the Army's physical fitness test, and I had a wife that loved me (probably too much because she did not mention that I had let myself go). Thus, I decided to make a change, and you might think that the first logical step is to commit to a diet. However, along my journey, I realized that starting a diet is not a great plan.

First, the term diet is mislabeled by society today. The "Diet" is merely the food we use to fuel our bodies. The act of eating food means we are all on a diet. The psychology of dieting also is designed to make us fail. As soon as we put a label on certain types of foods, we create a poor relationship with that food. There are no good or bad foods. There is only food. Some foods have more benefits than others. But who is to say the emotional benefit of the occasional scoop of ice cream (from happy, healthy cows of course) does not outweigh the health benefit of eating a salad every single day? Plus, as soon as we label something as "bad", and then we tell ourselves we cannot eat ice cream (or anything), the first thing we want is ice cream! So, what is the first thing we go for once we reach our goal weight? It is ice cream, and this time it is not a scoop we enjoy. This time we enjoy a full pint, or more. Then we enjoy another one the next day because we reached our goals, and we somehow find ourselves exactly where we started. Sometimes we end up at an even worse point. All because we decided ice cream is a "bad" food.

Not to mention, dieting is stressful. We feel like failures if we have a slip up. Then that slip up leads to a cascade of "cheating" because we already failed. Since we already failed, we may as well continue to fail is a common thought process among dieters with the all or nothing mentality. The term "cheat meal" also creates a poor psychological relationship with food. Anything not deemed perfectly healthy is "cheating", and failure and guilt become imminent. This all or nothing mentality is not the best way to live. Life is never all or nothing. Instead, it is the summation of all our choices ultimately leading to the person and place we are right now. Our health choices are the same way. Every meal is an opportunity for us to choose nutrient rich foods to help us reach our goals.

Too often, diets also restrict Calories to an unsustainable number. This creates a few problems. First, if we are not eating enough, we certainly are not getting enough essential nutrients our bodies need. Since most of us are already struggling to reach the right levels of nutrients from our diets due to lack of variety and diminished nutrient values in the food we do get, to shrink this number even more by restricting Calories could lead to huge health implications. Dr. Benjamin Bikman, a prominent researcher of insulin and its effects on health, put it like this on this Broken Brain Podcast (episode 154): imagine you are invited to a feast. This feast is filled with your favorite foods. A lot of money was spent, and you want to take advantage of it. In order to eat as much food as possible, what is a strategy you can implement to ensure this happens?

Eating Less and Exercise more. It is literally a strategy for gorging ourselves at a feast. Maybe we lose weight in the short term, but is it sustainable for long term results? Probably not. This strategy often leads to huge rebounds and what is commonly known as yo-yo dieting. We need to go beyond the advice of simply eating less and exercising more. That does not quite get us where we need to be.

Furthermore, severe Caloric restriction has been shown not to work. The body is pretty keen on keeping our weights where they are. There is a historic precedent to our bodies doing this. Our ancestors did not always know where their meals were going to come from. So, it makes sense to reason that our bodies evolved to keep weight on us in times of scarcity.

Then, there is the problem with all of the different types of diets. There are so many options out there: Atkins, Keto, Low-Carb, High-Carb, Zone, Vegan, South Beach, Mediterranean, Gluten Free, Raw Food....The list goes on. Each of these with plenty of people supporting them and swearing that they work. The amount of research on all these types of diets also varies. It is important to understand that each of us is different. Our genetic makeup has a big impact on whether these diets even work for us. Plus, maybe we are not ready mentally for these diets. It takes a lot of commitment to get into and maintain ketosis.

Many people get too caught up in the type of diet they used to get results, that they don't think that it was probably the act of cutting out processed foods and focusing on quality, nutrient dense foods that helped them reach their goals. If we all committed to this, we would reach most of our goals anyway!

So, what do we do? We need to create a healthy lifestyle. There is no doubt about that. Our focus should be on nutrient dense foods. These types of foods are going to be packed with nutrients and make us fuller. This is obviously important, but is that enough? Is simply eating healthy and moving more enough to get us to perform at our highest potential?   I would argue that it will not. In breaking down health, I came up with what I have begun to call "The Pillars of Health".

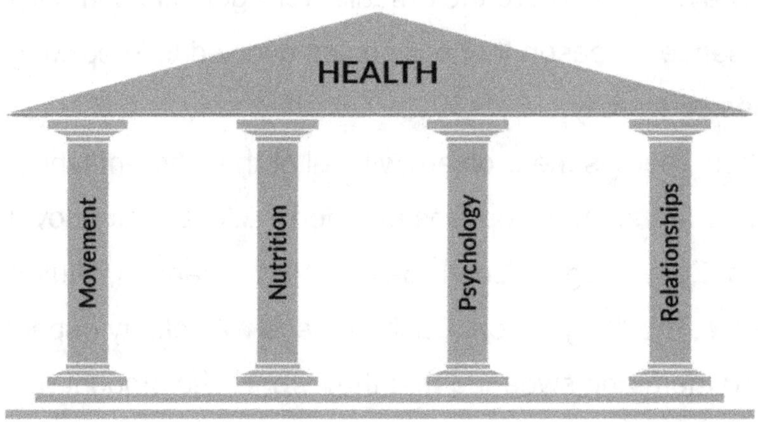

We have our obvious Pillars of Nutrition and Movement, and we will discuss those within the book for sure. But there are also the

Psychology and Relationship Pillars. These are both integral pieces of health and are a big reason why we do not actually dig into the science of food until the second section. Let us look at some different things that can positively impact each of the Pillars.

Movement

You have likely heard of the brain boosting benefits of movement. But how do we take full advantage of these benefits? There is an entire habit dedicated to movement. For now, understand the following:

- Move More - it really can be that simple. The fact of the matter is that Nutrition is going to weigh the heaviest on weight loss or weight gain. We will never out train a poor diet, so we should not use exercise as a punishment or a way to make up for not selecting food in line with our goals. Remember that Non-Exercise Activity Thermogenesis (NEAT) is a better way to increase Caloric Expenditure since we only exercise for about 60 minutes a day on training days.

- Exercise - that being said, there are still tremendous benefits to exercising. Be smart and start slowly. Hire a coach to help you progress properly. When done properly, exercise can help us feel better, move better, and increase our confidence. It also does not require as much as you might think.

- Recover - When we move more, our bodies need to recover. It is important we prioritize recovery just as much as we prioritize moving more. So, make sure to get plenty of sleep so the body can repair itself and get ready for the next day.

Nutrition

We know we need to eat better to be healthy, but what exactly does that look like? We will do a deeper dive into this in Section III. Here are some tips to help get things moving in the meantime:

- Focus on whole foods - it is less often the diet that brings results, and it is more often cutting processed foods. Do not get married to a specific style of eating, focus on whole foods and you will get closer to your goals.

- Quality not quantity - where our food comes from influences the effects it will have when we consume it. High quality food creates high quality reactions when consumed. We need to give our bodies the nutrients it needs.

- Eat for your goals - we are all as unique inside as we are outside, and our goals are very different as well. Our goals can help provide a road map when planning our food selection.

- Go to sleep - While we might not think about this first thing when it comes to nutrition, sleep has tremendous impacts on our hunger and fullness hormones. It is also a key time the body uses to detoxify. So, it is not enough to simply give the body the nutrients it needs. We must give it ample time to use those nutrients.

Psychology

The mind is a powerful tool when we set it up for success. However, we can also create an internal environment in which it could potentially take us further from our goals. Here are some key points for the Psychology Pillar:

- Set your Why - When our Why (the reason we do anything) is strong, it can serve as a lighthouse. It can guide our decisions. A strong why can help us make better decisions with how we spend our time, and who we spend our time with. When our decisions are in line with why, we feel a strong sense of purpose. Knowing why we do anything, makes us more productive and efficient, and it can even help us create a more positive outlook.

- Get outside - Nature is a powerful tool. Being outside in nature has been shown to have anti-depressive effects. Prioritize spending time outside. It may even be a good idea to exercise outside. This gives the brain boosting effects of exercise along with the brain boosting effects of nature. It is a win-win!

- Cut processed foods - we talked about this with the Nutrition Pillar. But this is how intricately linked each pillar is. By doing this, we can clear the brain fog and improve our cognition and mental capacity.

- Sleep - are you noticing the trend yet? Sleep allows us to recover emotionally and physically. When we get ample sleep, we are better prepared to handle the challenging emotional and cognitive tasks throughout the day. These capacities are limited, and sleep is when they can reset for the following day. It is also when we do much of our learning. So, go to sleep.

- Do not be afraid to seek help - there can be some negative associations with seeking mental help. However, we sometimes need help from a professional. They can help uncover things we may not even know are there. Like having a coach for any other aspect of our lives, a therapist can serve as a sort of mental coach. It takes strength to identify a problem and attack it head on. We only get one brain, so we need to take care of it!

Relationships

The people we surround ourselves with play a large part in our lives, and they can help propel us toward our goals or they can work against us and resist the change we are trying to achieve. There is an entire habit dedicated to this Pillar. For now, here are some key points:

- Set your support system - a strong support system keeps us on track. It also gives us a tribe that we belong to. We are tribal creatures, and we need a place where we feel we belong and can truly be ourselves. We help the people in this system, and they help us. This allows us to utilize the positive effects of serotonin and oxytocin - the cooperation hormones. If we do not have a support system that pushes us to grow and leaves us feeling recharged and ready to attack the day, it may be time to reevaluate the people we are spending our time with.

- Learn to love yourself - you are the number one person that you spend time with. So, when we barrage ourselves with negative self-talk, we can do much more harm than good. Be kind and forgiving to yourself. We do not expect others to be perfect all the time, and we should not expect that of ourselves either.

- Sleep - Sleep allows us to process our emotions and be less reactive when interacting with other people. It also restores our emotional intelligence. If you want to be a better friend, teammate, family member, or co-worker, it could be as easy as getting some more sleep.

By strengthening one pillar, we might notice the other Pillars solidifying as well. Where our minds go, the body will follow, and when the people around us understand our needs and desires, they are able to help push us forward. You may have noticed that there are things that impact all the Pillars. These Pillars are so intricately linked, that instead of breaking the book down into four separate sections, I decided on a habit-based approach that can help build up all the Pillars. Get any of these Pillars wrong and it will not take long to see our goals disappear into obscurity. It is my hope that this book will help you balance these Pillars. Once balanced, you have the foundations for health and performance ready to go where you dictate.

The Pillars were born as I tried to find areas in which I needed to improve to become a better coach. I worked to distill down the elements that I needed to be educate myself in order to help my athletes be successful, and I realized that these areas were areas in which we all need to balance if we are to be healthy. From there, I had the baseline of health in which success can be built. The only thing left was to structure a curriculum to cater to these Pillars. The habits are key elements that often get neglected in our culture, but they are paramount if we want to see long term success.

The most important thing is to understand that change does not happen overnight. Once we commit to a goal, we can design habits that start small and slowly build as we begin to master the habits and get closer to our overall goals. We cannot get caught up in labels of diets, or good or bad foods. We need to realize that each day we have choices and opportunities to get closer to our goals. However, that does not mean if we slip up one time we have failed. Instead, it just means that we are human. There is no shame in falling victim to the engineered foods containing mixtures of sugar and fats that are never found in nature. These products are designed to be addictive and keep us eating. Learn from the experience. Be kind to yourself. Practice forgiveness. Move on to the next opportunity. You got this.

Notes:

References

Asprey, D. (2018). *Game changers: What leaders, innovators, and mavericks do to win at life* HarperCollins.

Berardi, J., & Andrews, R. (2010). The essentials of sport and exercise nutrition. *Precision Nutrition 2013,*

Bubbs, M. (2019). *Peak: The new science of athletic performance that is revolutionizing sports* Chelsea Green Publishing.

Clear, J. (2018). *Atomic habits: An easy & proven way to build good habits & break bad ones* Avery.

Connolly, F., & White, P. (2017). *Game changer* Simon and Schuster
Coyle, D. (2018). *The culture code: The secrets of highly successful groups* Bantam.

Craft, L. L., & Perna, F. M. (2004). The benefits of exercise for the clinically depressed. *Primary Care Companion to the Journal of Clinical Psychiatry, 6*(3), 104.

Crockett, M. J., Clark, L., Lieberman, M. D., Tabibnia, G., & Robbins, T. W. (2010). Impulsive choice and altruistic punishment are correlated and increase in tandem with serotonin depletion. *Emotion, 10*(6), 855.

Dölen, G., Darvishzadeh, A., Huang, K. W., & Malenka, R. C. (2013). Social reward requires coordinated activity of nucleus accumbens oxytocin and serotonin. *Nature, 501*(7466), 179.

Gladwell, V. F., Brown, D. K., Wood, C., Sandercock, G. R., & Barton, J. L. (2013). The great outdoors: How a green exercise environment can benefit all. *Extreme Physiology & Medicine, 2*(1), 3.

Haff, G. G., & Triplett, N. T. (2015). *Essentials of strength training and conditioning 4th edition* Human kinetics.

Harari, Y. N. (2014). *Sapiens: A brief history of humankind* Random House.

https://www.precisionnutrition.com/diets-are-dead

http://main.poliquingroup.com/ArticlesMultimedia/Articles/Article/2793/Seven_Reasons_To_Never_Diet.aspx

Hyman, M. (2018). *Food: What the heck should I eat?* Hachette UK.

LaValle, J. B., & Yale, S. L. (2004). *Cracking the metabolic code: The nine keys to peak health* Basic Health Publications, Inc.

Learney, P. (2014). *N1 nutritional programming: The fundamentals of nutritional programming.* ACA.

Levine, J. A. (2002). Non-exercise activity thermogenesis (NEAT). *Best Practice & Research Clinical Endocrinology & Metabolism, 16*(4), 679-702.

Lunenburg, F. C. (2011). Goal-setting theory of motivation. *International Journal of Management, Business, and Administration, 15*(1), 1-6.

Purohit, D. (2020). *Broken Brain Podcast with Dhru Purohit. The Mind-Blowing Science of Fat-Burning and Insulin Resistance with Dr. Benjamin Bikman.* September 24, 2020 (154). https://open.spotify.com/show/7KXy3gx2FMFux1Hqiygh5g

Sapolsky, R. M. (2017). *Behave: The biology of humans at our best and worst* Penguin.

Schjerve, I. E., Tyldum, G. A., Tjønna, A. E., Stølen, T., Loennechen, J. P., Hansen, H. E., . . . Najjar, S. M. (2008). Both aerobic endurance and strength training programmes improve cardiovascular health in obese adults. *Clinical Science, 115*(9), 283-293.

Sinek, S. (2014). *Leaders eat last: Why some teams pull together and others don't* Penguin.

Taubes, G. (2007). *Good Calories Bad Calories.* Gary A. Knopf.

Walker, M. (2017). *Why we sleep: Unlocking the power of sleep and dreams* Simon and Schuster.

How to Use this Book

If you have ever asked me a question about training or nutrition, my answer was most likely "it depends" or "it's a tool". That is exactly how I view this book. It can be a great tool to help you develop the habits necessary to get the results you are looking for. However, it can also be a great paperweight (unless you are reading digitally). It is all in how you use it. It is not the end all be all of nutrition. In fact, it is fairly basic, and that is by design. I wanted it to be an introduction into nutrition. It was created for the average person to successfully reach their nutritional goals be it weight loss, healthier food choices, or even weight gain. However, it can also be used for athletes and high performers too. While there will be some subtle nuances into nutrition for maximizing high performance, the baseline of health is still critical. Without health, we cannot perform at any level in any arena or boardroom.

I choose a habit-based approach because it is hard to reach our goals. It requires work. There is no single tip or trick that anybody can give you to quickly reach your goals at a level that is sustainable. What is needed to get results is hard work and consistency in the basics. I also found it challenging to develop a method that focused on each pillar. In building the habits, I quickly noticed that many of the habits impact more than one pillar, and some even impact all four! As I mentioned earlier, they are not individual silos that work in isolation. They are complex systems of intricately linked processes that can work in our favor or our detriment. What is presented here is what I believe to be the basics that are required to reach a significant level of baseline health by building habits to grow all four Pillars of Health. So, this tool's value can only be assessed by you in how you use it to reach your potential.

When we embark on this life changing journey, we need to be held accountable (we will talk more about creating our support team later). If you are working through nutrition coaching with me, then you already have someone who is going to hold you accountable. Will someone else who sees you daily be able to hold you accountable? Absolutely! But having a coach to help guide you through this process is an invaluable tool. So, if you purchased this as a standalone tool, I highly recommend you get set up with a coach (CH Health & Fitness should definitely be your top choice, but I am biased). Head to https://www.coreyhobbs.com to sign up! If you are not near me or are not interested in working remotely, but still want to use this, then it is extremely pertinent that you find someone that is going to be able to hold you accountable. I mentioned Precision Nutrition earlier. They are the best in the game. So, I suggest finding someone that is certified by them to help you along your journey. That person also does not have to be a coach. It can be a friend you want to embark on this journey with. Like I mentioned earlier, you will get out of this tool whatever you put into it.

The goal is to provide enough science that you understand why each habit is important, but not so much that it bores you and scares you away from reading this. I get it, research studies and books can be intimidating. That's why I have tried to distill what I believe to be pertinent information to help you reach your goals mixed with a dash of science and evidence so that you understand that I'm not just making stuff up. The book may appear to be long, but there are many pages dedicated to notes and references. I promise that, for the most part, you will not have issues quickly reading through the habits so that you can begin to apply them as soon as you finish.

Before beginning, have a clear goal in mind of what you want to accomplish. Make it specific and give yourself plenty of time to reach it. Honestly, give yourself more time than you think. Remember that we are in this for long term health and results that are sustainable. Once you have your goal, figure out your why. Do not allow your why to be superficial. It needs to be deep and powerful. Get to the true root of why you want what you want. Once you have your initial why, continue to ask yourself why you think that why is important. Do this 5-6 times to really boil down what your why is. Then write it down. This is necessary because a strong why will help propel us forward when things inevitably get tough. Our why is always able to bring us back to our main goals and purpose. Next break down your goal into smaller goals. What steps need to be taken to reach those goals? Now break it down further. What actions are needed to make sure those smaller goals are accomplished? Break your goal down into the smallest imaginable processes and goals. Think about what you can today to accomplish your goals, and then what steps you would like to take this month, and even this year. There are always actionable steps we can take in the present moment to help us get towards our ultimate goals. Write them down and tell people too. It keeps us accountable and makes things a little more manageable when we see a clear path towards our goals. Now that we have small goals, they are much easier to obtain, and our success will release a rush of feel good hormones capable of propelling us towards our next goal. If you wrote them down, you could even cross them off a list giving you an even larger sense of accomplishment.

Goal Setting Checklist

- Write goals down
- Break goals down into smaller goals
- Focus on the Process
- Set reasonable time expectations
- Create the mindset of the person you want to be
- Know why

The book is broken down into habits (chapters). You may have noticed a section for notes after the previous chapter. Each habit will have a section at the end for notes. I also included some questions that may guide you in implementing each habit. This space is yours to record what you notice about the habit's impact on the way you eat, feel, or think. I recommend using it to record questions to bring up to your coach or accountability partner. It can also be a space where you do not do anything. Personally, I like taking notes at the end of a chapter, and I wanted you to have a place to record your thoughts and findings if you needed it. A plain old notebook or the margins work just as well too. The habits should be progressed slowly. It takes time to solidify these habits and make them part of our routines. The end of each habit will have a list of how to implement the habit if you want to take things slow, are looking for a little bit of a challenge, or you are ready to challenge yourself. Start wherever you and your coach are comfortable. A great way to assess which level to start at is something called "Ready, Willing, Able". Ask yourself, or have your coach ask you, how ready are you to complete this task? Then ask, how willing are you to complete this task? Finally, ask how able are you to complete this task? Rate each of these from a scale of 1-10. Once all 3 questions are a 9 or 10, that is where you should start the habit. Be honest with yourself. Just saying 9 or 10 because you know that is where you want to start is not a good strategy. Think critically and truly assess your answers to these questions. Once the habits become second nature, that is when we either make it more difficult, move on to the next habit, or both.

Some people will be able to move faster than others. The speed at which you go through the habits is not important. In fact, I strongly suggest you do not read ahead. Instead, I suggest taking at least 4 weeks with each individual habit. This is so the habit can truly become who you are. It will then be much easier to continue the old habits when moving on to the next one. What is important is the mastery of habits. There are a lot of habits. It will take a lot of time. There is no reason to rush. I told you earlier that real change is not instantaneous. It takes a significant contribution of time and effort.

So, take your time. Consistency and effort are going to be the keys to success. It may take over a year. Maybe even two, and that is okay. Learn to enjoy the process of improvement. Try to find little ways to improve daily and you will find yourself making consistent progress towards your goals. There are more ways to measure success than a number on a scale. How you feel, how you perform in other areas of life, and improved relationships are all improvements that have come forth from this type of coaching. Progress is progress. If you feel you need more or less difficulty, work with your coach to decide what the best plan of action for you is. Everyone is different. That is why I highly recommend you go through this with a coach.

No matter who you select to keep you accountable, it is imperative that you lay out clear expectations with them. It will help them give you what you need. With this approach, it is much more likely you both get what you need from this experience, and with clear expectations, the chance of either of you letting the other down is decreased. Honesty and openness are critical if we want to have a positive experience while being held accountable. In her book *Daring Greatly,* Brené Brown calls this "painting it done". With this strategy, paint a clear picture of what done looks like for both of you. It really helps clear up expectations for all parties involved. It also helps to streamline the communication process.

Each habit will also have a reference section. This is where you can see where the information provided to you is pulled from. I want to be completely transparent in where I am getting my information. But I also wanted you to be able to read things on your own if a particular subject really piqued your interest. Not all subjects will be interesting to everyone, but I encourage you to dive deeper into the subjects that interest you. As I mentioned earlier, I want to keep things as simple as possible, and this strategy allows me to do that. It is my hope that this book will serve as a tool that you can use repeatedly to hammer home the habits that are needed to strengthen and balance the Pillars of Health. So, without further ado, let us get started.

Notes

What are your goals, and what is your timeframe for reaching your goals?

What is your Why?

Who is holding you accountable? Have you been clear with your expectations of them?

References

Berardi, J., & Andrews, R. (2010). *The essentials of sport and exercise nutrition*. Precision Nutrition.

Brown, B. (2018). *Dare to Lead: Brave Work. Tough Conversations. Whole Hearts*. Random House.

Clear, J. (2018). Atomic habits: An easy & proven way to build good habits & break bad ones Avery.

Lunenburg, F. C. (2011). Goal-setting theory of motivation. *International Journal of Management, Business, and Administration, 15*(1), 1-6.

Sinek, S. (2009). *Start with why: How great leaders inspire everyone to take action* Penguin.

33

Section II: Before the Food

Before we even begin to talk about food, there is actually a few things we need to get in order first. These first couple of habits are designed to build from one another and cascade into an overflowing river of success. Sounds a little dramatic, but these first few habits really can be the deciding factor in success.

Habit 1: Make Time

I know what you're probably thinking: "Corey, what the heck? I thought this was a Nutrition book!". Take a deep breath. Perfect. As I mentioned earlier, this book is designed to help you create the habits necessary for you to reach your goals. So, before we even talk about what we are eating, we need to get our bodies and minds in order first. For, where the mind goes, the body will follow.

Life today is nonstop. Our schedules are packed with meetings, our children are playing sports or hanging with friends, and then we want to be able to spend time with our friends and socialize too. Many of us do not even step away from our desks to eat lunch at work, and dinners are often spent in front of the TV. If we do not learn how to make time for ourselves and our goals, it will be difficult to implement the rest of the habits. Once we have this habit down, it becomes less challenging to implement the more difficult habits because we already are prioritizing our health and our goals.

Our lives are filled with constant stressors that we did not have thousands of years ago. Our lifestyles are so different that the diseases that plague society today are not the same as those that plagued our ancestors. Our ancestors constantly worried about whether or not they would be mauled by a sabretooth tiger. Some of our biggest stressors are our jobs, families, and friends. Even something as simple as sitting in traffic can be a stressor. We are also highly individual. Sitting in traffic may be a stressor for you, but it does not bother me at all. These stressors we face every day, but a sabretooth tiger was not likely to threaten our ancestors every single day. What is worse, is that our bodies cannot tell the difference between the stress of our jobs, families, or friends and that from the threat of a predator. So, it reacts in the exact same way for both situations. It does this despite the fact that our lives are rarely ever actually in danger. When our bodies are constantly in a stress response state, they can cause serious harm to themselves.

In his book, *Why Zebras Do Not Get Ulcers*, Dr. Robert Sapolsky chronicles the difference between the chronic stressors of humans and Zebras. He begins with, "...stress can make us sick, and a critical shift in medicine has been the recognition that many of the damaging diseases of slow accumulation can be either caused or made worse by stress." Science has shown that chronic levels of elevated stress have links to heart disease, metabolic syndrome, and impaired cognition to just name a few.

So, why does this happen? The stress response is a tool the body has created to respond to acute events. It is great for running away from that sabretooth tiger and keeping us alive. However, it is not great when it is activated daily in response to our bosses, finances, or relationships. Many of the dangers we face today are those which we create in our heads. That exam is not going to kill us, and our boss is not likely to kill us if we miss a deadline either.

Anything can be a stressor, and the stress response can even be activated in anticipation of something that we worry might happen. Therefore, the perception of a stressor is also critical. If we do not think of something as a stressor, we will not have the effects of stress. This is the exact reason that I am able to sit in traffic without being stressed, and you may feel your blood boiling when you are in the exact same situation. If we think of something as a stressor, we will receive a stress response. Which means we actually have some power in how we respond to situations. There are numerous factors we cannot control. The actions of other people for example, but our own actions and thoughts are always within our control.

Why is the stress response bad? It is not. Our bodies need stressors to grow and adapt to situations to make us more likely to survive. The stress response diverts blood flow from our organs and shuts down digestion. It floods our bodies with excitatory hormones like adrenaline. These things are all great in small doses when we need them. Over time, chronic stress can cause digestive distress, insomnia, increased inflammation, and impaired immune function. So, we cannot absorb the nutrients we are eating, our bodies cannot repair during sleep, and we are at a higher risk of getting sick. All these factors just continue the cycle of disease making us continue to get worse despite our best efforts.

All these actions are controlled by our sympathetic nervous system. It is more commonly known as our "fight or flight" system. We are not always fighting, so we do not always need this system activated in our bodies. Instead, we need our parasympathetic nervous system activated. This system is more commonly known as our "rest and digest" system. We need this system to be functioning properly. As its name suggests, it is critical for recovery and absorption of the nutrients we take in. We need our parasympathetic nervous system functioning properly so that our gastrointestinal tract (GI Tract) functions properly. The GI tract is responsible for the digestion and absorption of the nutrients we take in. It also contains the enteric nervous system, sometimes called our second brain because it secretes neurotransmitters and hormones that are responsible for many of the processes within the body. For example, 80% of the serotonin created within the body comes from the enteric nervous system.

But the GI tract does not handle digestion and absorption alone. Our GI tracts are filled with bacteria. Some of them are good, and some of them are bad. These bacteria actually assist in the breaking down of what we eat. When we give our bodies the nutrients it needs and wants, the good bacteria can flourish, and the bad bacteria are kept at bay. However, when we do not give our bodies the nutrients it needs, the bad bacteria can take over. They thrive on highly processed foods. They also thrive in the acidic environment within our bodies chronic stress creates. We need our good bacteria working with our bodies because they also create some of the neurotransmitters our bodies use.

Put simply, the sympathetic nervous system is great if we are about to wrestle our little brother. Our brains work faster, our muscles perform optimally, and our bodies are ready to dominate our opponent at the task at hand. However, once we are done, we go back to being siblings and not enemies (in many cases). For our bodies to function optimally, we need to be able to stop relying on that fight or flight system and allow our rest and digest system to take over. This is where our first habit comes into play. We need to make time for ourselves.

The saying that we cannot pour from an empty cup is an overused troupe that we understand, but rarely apply. So, let us take it literally for a moment to truly understand why this is important. You are thirsty. I know you are because I told you are. Even if you are not, work with me here. So, since you are thirsty you need to drink water. Pretty simple problem with a simple solution. You get up and go to the cupboard to grab 2 cups. One for pouring, and one for drinking. Go ahead and designate one of those cups for drinking and one for pouring. Now, take your pouring cup and pour its contents into the drinking cup. What happened? Unless you are some sort of wizard, absolutely nothing happened.

Now, take your pouring cup and fill it with water. Pour the contents of the pouring cup into your drinking cup. What happened this time? The water was poured from one cup to the other, and this time there was no wizardry required. We are pouring cups. We likely have plenty of people working to take our contents (energy) so that they can replenish their own thirst (whatever they need from us). These people are stressors. Whether we recognize them as such or not. Our kids are stressors, our spouses are stressors, our friends are stressors. Somewhere down the line, we run out of water to pour into other people. There is even a name for this phenomenon. It is called Compassion Fatigue. Continuing to put others before ourselves without having an outlet for our own issues drains our time and energy. Pair that with the stress of constantly being bombarded by social media and the "perfect" lives of those we follow, we have a recipe for disaster. The sympathetic nervous system works tirelessly to empty our cups, and the parasympathetic nervous system works to replenish it. This is why it is so critical to make time for ourselves.

We need to fill our cups. How do we do it? There are many ways we can take time for ourselves to replenish our cups. How we do it is going to depend highly on the individual. The first thing is being open about the fact that we need time to ourselves. When we pretend that everything is alright, we build more stress into our already overstressed lives. The sole act of admitting we are stressed and overwhelmed can lift a huge burden. The best part is that humans are designed to be compassionate creatures. In fact, as a species, we never could have made it this far without being willing to help those in need. So, when we admit we need help, people often jump at the opportunity to give us assistance.

Next, we need to be able to say no. No is a tremendous tool in giving us the power back in our lives. Sometimes there are things we just do not want to do. While there are moments in which we do need to suck it up and push through, most of the time we are completely in control of what we do or do not give our time to. If an activity does not directly bring joy or work to advance any goals we have in place, we should say no. Yes, people will be disappointed. But, if we are open with them about why we are saying no, that we just need time to ourselves, they will usually understand. If they do not, it may be time to create a new circle of influence. We will talk more about that in a few chapters.

We have cleared up our schedules, we have said no, and we no longer have jam packed calendar with every minute accounted for. What do we do next? Anything! The criteria for saying no above was whether something brought joy or helped with goals we had. These same criteria can be used to dictate how we use the extra time we have created. Perhaps you need time with your significant other to show your appreciation and love with a special night out. Perfect. Or maybe there is a book or movie you have been meaning to catch up on. Now is the time for that too. The key is being comfortable with being with ourselves. We can also start to list and name things we are grateful for. Focusing on the things we are grateful for allows us to be reminded of the good things in our lives instead of all the things that are not going the way we planned. To start, we may need a reminder in our calendar to tell us to take this time. That is okay. After the reminder, put the phone down and be in the present moment. Maybe take some time to journal or be reminded of all there is to be grateful for (you can even practice in the notes section). Once we do that, we can work on activating the parasympathetic nervous system to really get our cups refilled.

Here is a trick that only takes 5 minutes and is a great way to get into that rest and digest state. Lie flat on your belly with your head on top of your hands and eyes closed. Take a long inhale through your nose, pause, take a long, forceful exhale through your mouth, and pause again. Repeat this until the 5 minutes have passed. Work to get your inhale to 4 seconds and your exhale to 8 seconds. That is it. Even if you cannot clear your schedule, this 5-minute exercise is a great way to calm nerves and relieve stress. Of course, you can always do it for longer, and you do not even need to be lying down to do it either. It can be done seated or even driving. Although you might want to skip the eyes closed part if you are driving.

Make Time

Now that we have an idea of why it is important to make time, we can get into how to implement the habit. The trick is to find what works best for you. We are all highly individual. I cannot tell you what is going to be best in your situation. That is something you must find on your own. A coach can help brainstorm ideas, but the execution falls on you. Use the notes section to brainstorm and track how different strategies work for you, and then work with your coach or accountability partner to really dial in what your best practice might be. Focus on this habit for the next 4 weeks. Take more time if you need. Remember, we truly want this to become part of our lives.

- Starting Slow - 1-2 days a week schedule at least 5 minutes for yourself. It can be anything, but it cannot be work or anything else that might stress you out. The breathing drill discussed above is a great start for this quick habit. Work to increase the time spent for yourself as well as how many days you do it. Add either time or days. Try not to do both. By doing too much too soon we run the risk of getting overwhelmed.

- A Little More Challenging - Every day of the week schedule at least 15 minutes for yourself. Same rules as above. Start reminding yourself of everything there is to be grateful for in your life.

- Ready for a Challenge - Every day of the week, take 30-60 minutes for yourself. This is a great time to start experimenting with a new hobby, journaling, or even meditation.

Notes

General notes about the habit:

How are you planning on implementing this habit?

How ready, willing, and able are you to implement your strategy? (for a reminder on how to use this activity, see page 28)

What are some potential roadblocks you may face?

What are some strategies you can use prepare for these roadblocks?

What have you noticed about how you feel, think, or act after implementing this habit?

Which Pillars do you feel that this habit impacts? Why?

Any questions, comments, or concerns to bring up with your coach?

References

Berardi, J., & Andrews, R. (2010). *The essentials of sport and exercise nutrition.* Precision Nutrition.

Bubbs, M. (2019). *Peak: The new science of athletic performance that is revolutionizing sports* Chelsea Green Publishing.

Connolly, F., & White, P. (2017). *Game changer* Simon and Schuster.

Figley, C. R. (2002). Compassion fatigue: Psychotherapists' chronic lack of self-care. *Journal of Clinical Psychology, 58*(11), 1433-1441.

Harari, Y. N. (2014). *Sapiens: A brief history of humankind* Random House.

Sapolsky, R. M. (2004). *Why zebras do not get ulcers: The acclaimed guide to stress, stress-related diseases, and coping-now revised and updated* Holt paperbacks.

Vitaliano, P. P., Scanlan, J. M., Zhang, J., Savage, M. V., Hirsch, I. B., & Siegler, I. C. (2002). A path model of chronic stress, the metabolic syndrome, and coronary heart disease. *Psychosomatic Medicine, 64*(3), 418-435.

Habit 2: Slow Down

This habit may seem similar to the first. But, instead of things going on around us, this refers to how we eat our food. I strongly believe that even if you take nothing else from this book and stop after this chapter, these first two habits have enough power behind them that you could make a strong advance towards your goals. To start, we will give a brief rundown on how digestion happens, and then get into why slowing down is such a critical skill. Just a note, this is likely the only habit where if your goal is to gain weight, you can skip it. Simply work with your coach to find a strategy better suited to your needs.

We learned a bit about the GI tract earlier, and we will get into a little more detail here. But this is still a basic breakdown of what happens. The references at the end of the chapter can give some deeper insight into what is happening within our bodies if you need more.

Believe it or not, the digestion process happens before food even enters our bodies. The simple act of thinking of or smelling food can begin the digestive process. When our mouths start watering after smelling our food, that is our bodies getting ready to digest the food we are about to eat. Once the food is in our mouths we begin chewing. This a super important step that many of us glance over. We are busy, so we rush through our meals chewing minimally. In the book, *Game Changer: The Art of Sport Science,* Dr. Fergus Connolly eloquently notes that the stomach has no teeth. So, we must help our stomachs by breaking down food as much as possible through chewing. The more we can break down before food enters the stomach, the better our entire digestive system will be able to function.

After we finish chewing our food, bolus is formed. Bolus is just a fancy name for chewed food. We swallow the bolus, and it enters our esophagus. The esophagus does little to aid in digestion. Its main purpose is to move food into the stomach. There is also a ring like muscle called the lower esophageal sphincter which prevents stomach acid from rising back into our throats and mouths which is commonly known as GERD (gastroesophageal reflux disease). There are numerous factors which affect GERD, so if you're experiencing burning in the back of your throat, nausea and vomiting, pressure/pain in the chest, bloating and burping, and sometimes tooth erosion, there are a few things you can try. Eat slowly, eat smaller meals, focus on whole foods, or use a food journal to see if there is a link between what you eat and when the symptoms arise. Should the problem persist, you should see your doctor and try to get the root cause of the matter.

Once in the stomach, the bolus mixes with stomach acid to produce chyme. There are a few things which can be absorbed in the stomach such as some drugs, water, some vitamins, alcohol, and certain short chain fatty acids. From here the chyme begins to enter the small intestine. This process takes between 1 and 4 hours depending on the contents of the meal. Carbohydrates empty the fastest. Protein is next in line, and fats are the last to move through. Liquids move quicker than solids, and smaller particles will move more quickly than their larger counterparts.

Once in the small intestines, it takes 4-8 hours for the chyme to completely move through. The slow movement gives our small intestines optimal time to absorb all the nutrients we have ingested. From here, the remaining food moves into the large intestines. Some nutrients will head to the liver for processing, and the rest moves into the large intestine. The liver is one of the body's main detoxifiers, but it also helps to further break down fats, proteins, and carbohydrates so the body can properly utilize them. It is estimated that we process 60 tons of food in our lifetimes. This means our digestion and detoxifying systems are quite busy. We should reduce the burden on these systems from heavy metals, pesticides, fertilizers, and other contaminants by working to get the highest quality food we can.

The large intestine is responsible for absorbing some leftovers and moving the stuff we do not want to get ready to be excreted. Anything not absorbed will be secreted through feces or urine. Within the large intestines, the food will likely stay for 12-25 hours. It is interesting to note that the length of the intestines determines the food an animal can eat and digest. For example, meat eaters will have longer small intestines and shorter large intestines. Plant eaters have the opposite. Humans land somewhere between the two and can absorb and digest a good mixture of foods.

Bacteria also play a role in the digestion of the foods we eat. Bacteria work by helping our bodies break down and absorb the things it cannot break down on its own, such as fiber. Keeping our bacteria healthy can play a large role in several bodily functions to include regulating inflammation, regulating our mood and nervous system function, regulating hormones throughout the body, and regulating our body composition to name only a few. Things such as antibiotics can disrupt the natural system within our guts. So, it is important to eat, or potentially supplement, prebiotic and probiotic foods which support the growth of healthy bacteria within our guts. Some of these foods include sauerkraut, yogurt, or kefir. Just be careful as some of these when bought in stores have additives that are not great for our bodies such as extra sugar.

Now that we have a basic understanding of how the digestive process works, we should talk about a couple of the things that might disrupt the process. The first one we talked about with the previous habit and is why it is so critical to have that habit down before moving on: Stress. In high stress environments, our bodies cannot properly digest foods. As a quick recap, the sympathetic nervous system diverts blood from our digestive organs to those critical to our survival. Thus, we need to ensure we know how to activate our parasympathetic nervous system to rest and digest. Eating too quickly can also disrupt the process because our food is not broken down enough when the food gets to our stomachs. Remember, the stomach does not have teeth. We must help it out as much as we can. We can help it by ensuring it is getting enough blood and nutrients to do its job (activating parasympathetic nervous system) and chewing our food (slowing down).

Throughout this entire process there are many digestive enzymes and hormones that play large roles in helping our bodies absorb the food we ingest. However, there are 2 enzymes that are particularly critical to our hunger: Leptin and Ghrelin. These hormones influence our internal drive to eat more or less.

Leptin is secreted mainly by fat cells. So, its main purpose is energy balance within the body. Leptin lets our body know that it is well fed and does not need any additional food. Thus, when our energy levels are adequate, leptin will be high, and when our energy levels are inadequate, our leptin levels will be low. Leptin can be disrupted by activation of the sympathetic nervous system as well.

Ghrelin is released by several cells throughout the body, and it acts directly on the brain. It is used to signal that energy levels are too low. It then goes down after ingesting a meal.

The crucial part of these signaling hormones is that they do not act instantaneously. They take about 15-20 minutes to adequately signal to the body that it has enough energy flowing throughout it. That is why it is not a good idea to wait to eat until we are "starving", go on overly restrictive diets, or rush through meals. They are also impacted significantly by sleep (which we will talk more about shortly) and stress. If these hormones are not balanced or signaling to the body what it needs, overeating can rapidly descend on us. We often will not even recognize increased consumption due to imbalanced hormones while it is happening.

Therefore, slowing down and being mindful when we are eating is so critical. It could be the difference in eating the right amount of food in the right proportions and too much food in inadequate proportions. Luckily, there are some steps we can take to make sure these hormones can work the way they are supposed to.

We also need to notice if we are hungry or eating for another reason such as boredom, thirst, or a social situation where food is simply present. By slowing down, we can truly understand and feel what hunger and satiety feel like. Start to notice if you are eating in situations where you are not actually hungry. What is the trigger? The simple act of noticing these things can help us reduce the amount of times it happens. Slow down and be present. Try to understand what your body is telling you it needs. You may even begin to notice that we are able to thrive on much less food than we think.

The first trick we can use is avoiding distractions while we eat. Put the phone down, get away from your desk, turn the TV off, and pay attention to your meal. Notice the different flavors present. How do you feel after the meal? Can you name every ingredient you taste? Distracted eating is a great way to overconsume. When eat mindlessly, we may not notice our fullness cues. So, put the distractions away and enjoy your meal. Work, the tv, and your phone will all still be there when you are finished.

Another trick is setting a timer for our meals. Simply set a timer and try not to finish the meal before the time runs out. Start with something easy like 5-6 minutes and add time the more comfortable you get with it. Make it fun and something you want to do. This way, you are more likely to stick with it as time is added.

The simple act of putting silverware down between bites is also a great tool. It is hard to inhale food rapidly if after each bite we need to pick up the fork or spoon.

Have a conversation with those around you. Enjoy their presence and their company. Talk about how the food tastes, how your days were, or any other topic. Just take the time to be with the people around you and notice how eating naturally slows down.

Try to get to 40-50 chews per bite of food. It is difficult to do this rapidly, and it is also difficult to not break down your food enough when using this technique. This should allow you to breakdown your food plenty before it enters the stomach.

You can also combine any or all of these too. Again, it is all about finding out what works best for you in your situation. Try a few or come up with different techniques on your own. Notice how you feel when you slow down. You might notice you eat less food, but still get full.

Slow Down

Now that we have an idea of why it is important to slow down, we can get into how to implement the habit. The trick is to find what works best for you. We are all highly individual. I cannot tell you what is going to be best in your situation. That is something you must find on your own. A coach can help brainstorm ideas, but the execution falls on you. Use the notes section to brainstorm and track how different strategies work for you, and then work with your coach or accountability partner to really dial in what your best practice might be. Do not forget to continue the previous habit because it all works together. Focus on this habit for the next 4 weeks. Take more time if you need. Remember, we truly want this to become part of our lives.

- Start Slow - Pick a single meal one day a week. Use one of the techniques above to really slow down and be mindful of what you are eating. Notice how the food tastes and how you feel while eating it.

- A Little More Challenging - Pick a couple of meals a few days a week. Utilize the same strategy as above. Start to notice if you are eating due to things other than hunger

- Ready for a Challenge - Utilize the above strategies at every meal. Make sure you are only eating when you are actually hungry.

Notes

General notes about the habit:

How are you planning on implementing this habit?

How ready, willing, and able are you to implement your strategy? (for a reminder on how to use this activity, see page 28)

What are some potential roadblocks you may face?

What are some strategies you can use prepare for these roadblocks?

What have you noticed about how you feel, think, or act after implementing this habit?

Which Pillars do you feel that this habit impacts? Why?

Any questions, comments, or concerns to bring up with your coach?

References

Berardi, J., & Andrews, R. (2010). *The essentials of sport and exercise nutrition.* Precision Nutrition.

Connolly, F., & White, P. (2017). *Game changer* Simon and Schuster.

Klok, M. D., Jakobsdottir, S., & Drent, M. L. (2007). The role of leptin and ghrelin in the regulation of food intake and body weight in humans: A review. *Obesity Reviews, 8*(1), 21-34.

Luna, R. A., & Foster, J. A. (2015). Gut brain axis: Diet microbiota interactions and implications for modulation of anxiety and depression. *Current Opinion in Biotechnology, 32*, 35-41.

Taheri, S., Lin, L., Austin, D., Young, T., & Mignot, E. (2004). Short sleep duration is associated with reduced leptin, elevated ghrelin, and increased body mass index. *PLoS Medicine, 1*(3), e62.

Habit 3: Go to Sleep

Sleep is one of the easiest ways to enhance performance, but the last thing people want to use to their advantage. In fact, in his book *Why We Sleep: Unlocking the Power of Sleep and Dreams* Dr. Matthew Walker points out on the very first page that two thirds of adults in all of the developed nations do not get the recommended amount of sleep. We consistently highlight and praise "the grind". However, the grind causes much more damage than good. Dr. Walker continues, "routinely sleeping less than six or seven hours a night demolishes your immune system, more than doubling your risk of cancer." Sleep is free and has several health boosting benefits when we make the time to get enough of it. Sleep is responsible for resetting our emotional response mechanisms, clearing toxins from the brain, enhancing learning, improving hormone secretion, and many other important functions. A lack of sleep has been linked to depressed immune function, reduced emotional capacity, reduced cognitive function, metabolic disease, and obesity.

In fact, a lack of sleep can even be the reason we cannot seem to get our body composition the way we want it. Remember those two hormones we talked about with the last habit? Leptin and Ghrelin are highly impacted by sleep. When we get enough, these two hormones are able to act appropriately. However, when we do not get enough sleep, these two hormones get out of synch which can seriously impact how we feel hunger. To put it quite simply, we feel hungrier frequently, and cannot seem to ever get full. You have probably even felt this before. Have you ever stayed up later than normal to watch a movie or binge a show? Did you notice that you were more hungry than usual, and you could not seem to stop snacking? That is what happens when we do not get enough sleep and Leptin and Ghrelin become out of synch with our body's normal rhythm. It is not difficult to see how consistently not getting enough sleep can eventually lead to obesity and the plethora of health-related issues that come with it.

It is not just body composition that is affected by sleep either. During sleep the brain moves memories from a short-term storage to a long-term storage area. It also creates links to abstract memories enhancing creativity and the ability to solve complex problems with creative solutions. Sleep enhances the ability to recall what we have learned, and this happens several days after learning. So, if we get great sleep right after learning something, but stay up late 2 or 3 nights later, memory is likely to decay. Sleep also enhances our motor control (think muscle memory) in a similar way. Which is why we might practice something all day, but never master the tasks only to come back after a good night of restful sleep completing the skill with ease.

Sleep even enhances immune function. A lack of sleep leaves the sympathetic nervous system (fight or flight) in the "on" position. This increases the hormone production of hormones like epinephrine and cortisol. These hormones themselves are not dangerous but if elevated chronically can leave our bodies Inflamed and hinder the body's immune response. These responses begin to show after even one night of sleep deprivation! If we are sick and inflamed, we are not going to train well, and we certainly are not going to work efficiently. Hormones such as Growth Hormone and Testosterone are also released in large quantities during sleep. To make matters worse, a lack of sleep decreases aerobic performance and power output! So, if you are not seeing any gains in the gym or cannot seem to lose those couple of pounds despite eating perfectly instead of trying to add more supplements to your stack, reach for a pillow. It is much cheaper, and odds are it will do more for you.

Detoxification is a crucial process that occurs during sleep. The brain has cells called glial cells which are part of the glymphatic system (think the brain's lymph system or the bodyguard for the brain). These cells attach to toxins in the brain and shrink them down so that they can be removed. They are basically a trash compactor for your brain. One important protein these cells remove is the Amyloid protein which has a critical link to Alzheimer's. But these cells only do this while we sleep. Many Psychiatric conditions are also accompanied by a sleep disorder. This could raise the question of whether the psychiatric issue caused the sleep disorder, or perhaps the sleep disorder caused the psychiatric issue?

When we miss sleep, productivity drops. Thus, we need to work longer to complete the tasks required of us. Since we now need to work longer, we are likely to stay up later and wake up at the same time perpetuating the cycle of sleep deprivation. Furthermore, the part of the brain responsible for self-control and emotional impulse control (emotional IQ), the frontal lobe, is turned off when there is a lack of sleep present. With a reduced emotional IQ, we lose awareness for ourselves and make it harder to collaborate with those around us. Sleep deprivation is killing your team. So, not only are we working longer, slower and making worse decisions, but we are also not coming up with creative solutions or collaborating with our coworkers. Thus, a lack of sleep creates a cyclical effect of poor performance regardless of the domain.

Sleep is also crucial during the early stages of life. It is a driving force of brain maturation. This is why babies sleep so much. But this does not just apply to babies. Our children need plenty of sleep too. This is the prime time for brain building and development. Unfortunately, early school start times are hindering this development. School start times are based on the circadian rhythms of adults, but our circadian rhythms change throughout our lives. When a child needs to sleep is quite different than us as adults. This could very likely why our "lazy" teenagers seem so unproductive. The teenage years have a shift of circadian rhythm which keeps them up later but requires them to sleep in more. So, maybe they are not so lazy after all.

This does not just apply to kids and teenagers either. We are all different with our circadian rhythms. Dr. Michael Breus notes in *The Power of When* that there are four distinct chronotypes that we see as adults. Our chronotypes determine when we are most productive, or when we are best suited for sleep. For example, I am a Bear chronotype. I am most productive in the morning, and my productivity wanes as the day progresses. To find out about your chronotype, head to www.thepowerofwhenquiz.com. In a perfect world, we would be able to create our schedules to match our productivity levels. But, if we have less of a say in our actual work schedules, we may be able to use this information to schedule our day that will allow us to put forth a high quality of work.

Unfortunately, we can never "make up" sleep. Once sleep is missed, it is missed for good. There is no sleep bank where we can save up a bunch on the weekends and make withdrawals during the week when we "need" to sleep less. There will always be work to do, but most of the time it is not a life or death matter. Work will always be there in the morning.

There are several things that will negatively impact sleep we should all be aware of. The first is alcohol. We have heard of a nightcap, but that probably is not in our best interest. Alcohol will work well to put you to sleep. However, the body has to work very hard to clear the alcohol from the system, so while the drive to sleep is increased while drinking, the sleep that occurs is more like a coma (this is actually the case when you take sleep aiding drugs as well which is why you may not feel like you got any rest following a night on sleep aids, because you didn't). To take it a step further, we often wake up when the body is working to clear the toxins. I am sure you can recall a night or early morning after drinking where you just cannot get back to sleep. That is caused by the body working to get back to normal. This is not to steer you away from alcohol. But merely information so that you can make the best choices to help you reach your goals. Trust me, I am all about enjoying a night out with good friends enjoying some alcoholic drinks! Context is king.

Stress also can negatively impact sleep. We learned earlier how our sympathetic nervous system works to keep us alive in high threat situations. Well, if our body thinks it is in danger, it will not want to allow restful sleep to occur. This is why we may struggle to sleep the night before a big performance or exam, and it is also why it is so important to learn how to activate our parasympathetic nervous system so that we can properly rest and recover.

Blue light, the light emitted by electronic screens, light in general while sleeping, noise, late caffeine consumption, exercising too close to bedtime, and movement (think pets) are also things that might impact our sleep. We will go over some tips to maximize our sleep in the coming pages, so do not get too worried.

As a society we should no longer glorify "the grind" and the "I'll sleep when I'm dead" mentality. Our praise should go to the individuals prioritizing their health and working consistently to ensure they are taking the necessary steps to maintain proper habits to better serve others. A lack of sleep is not something that should be taken lightly. There will be situations where adequate sleep just is not in the cards (my newborn has shown that to me). However, we should do everything we can to take steps to maximize our sleep.

The good news is there are plenty of steps we can take to ensure we are getting the best sleep possible. If you are having issues sleeping, or want to maximize the time spent sleeping, start to practice proper sleep hygiene. Sleep in a pitch-black room, you should not even be able to see your hand in front of your face. Keep the temperature cool around 65-67 degrees Fahrenheit. Eliminate screen time about 90-120 minutes before bedtime. Wind down, try writing in a journal or deep breathing prior to bed to increase parasympathetic tone. Avoid caffeine in the afternoon. Exercise, but avoid exercise 2 hours before bed. Go to bed before 11, the time you are asleep matters just as much as the time spent asleep. You can also try to schedule all your work according to your circadian rhythm. Track your sleep. There are several apps and products out there that do this for you. I have an Oura ring, and it gives me great information on my sleep. However, smart watches and other sleep trackers such as whoop, Apple Watch, etc. are also great tools. A simple sleep journal will also do the trick. Use the notes section to track what things might impact how you sleep either positively or negatively. It can also be used to track how more sleep changes your performance throughout the day.

If you truly feel that you are doing everything right and you still feel fatigued upon waking, it may be necessary to schedule a sleep test. You might be plagued by sleep apnea in which a lack of oxygen is forcing you to wake up several times throughout the night. If this test comes back negative, you may have an issue with jaw shape which causes pressure to build within your airways while you sleep. This is often accompanied by a dry mouth. Depending on the severity, a mouthguard or even surgery may be necessary to as a permanent solution.

Go to Sleep

Now that we have an idea of why it is important to go to sleep, we can get into how to implement the habit. The trick is to find what works best for you. We are all highly individual. I cannot tell you what is going to be best in your situation. That is something you must find on your own. A coach can help brainstorm ideas, but the execution falls on you. Use the notes section to brainstorm and track how different strategies work for you, and then work with your coach or accountability partner to really dial in what your best practice might be. Do not forget to continue the previous habits because they all work together. Focus on this habit for the next 4 weeks. Take more time if you need. Remember, we truly want this to become part of our lives.

- Take it Slow - Try to get 30 extra minutes of sleep a few times a week. Try to find things that positively or negatively impact how you sleep.

- A Little More Challenging - Add 30 minutes to an hour of extra sleep every night of the week. Track how the extra sleep impacts your mood and performance.

- Ready for a Challenge - get at least 8 hours of sleep every night of the week. Try to match your sleep with your chronotype. Track your performance and how different things might impact your sleep positively or negatively.

Notes

General notes about the habit:

How are you planning on implementing this habit?

How ready, willing, and able are you to implement your strategy? (for a reminder on how to use this activity, see page 28)

What are some potential roadblocks you may face?

What are some strategies you can use prepare for these roadblocks?

What have you noticed about how you feel, think, or act after implementing this habit?

Which Pillars do you feel that this habit impacts? Why?

Any questions, comments, or concerns to bring up with your coach?

References

Berardi, J., & Andrews, R. (2010). *The essentials of sport and exercise nutrition.* Precision Nutrition.

Bubbs, M. (2019). *Peak: The new science of athletic performance that is revolutionizing sports* Chelsea Green Publishing.

Connolly, F., & White, P. (2017). *Game changer* Simon and Schuster.

https://blog.designsforhealth.com/teenagers-insufficient-sleep-obesity-gotosleep

https://blog.designsforhealth.com/Insulin%20Sensitivity%20and%20Sleep%2C%20or%20Lack%20Thereof

https://blog.bulletproof.com/how-to-hack-your-sleep-the-art-and-science-of-sleeping

https://www.thepowerofwhenquiz.com

Sapolsky, R. M. (2004). *Why zebras do not get ulcers: The acclaimed guide to stress, stress-related diseases, and coping-now revised and updated* Holt paperbacks.

Taheri, S., Lin, L., Austin, D., Young, T., & Mignot, E. (2004). Short sleep duration is associated with reduced leptin, elevated ghrelin, and increased body mass index. *PLoS Medicine, 1*(3), e62.

Verstegen, M., & Williams, P. (2014). *Every day is game day: Train like the pros with a no-holds-barred exercise and nutrition plan for peak performance* Penguin.

Walker, M. (2017). *Why we sleep: Unlocking the power of sleep and dreams* Simon and Schuster.

Habit 4: Build your Supporting Cast

Jim Rohn, an entrepreneur and motivational speaker, is known for many of his quotes and his advice. One that you might immediately recognize is that we are the product of the 5 people we spend most of our time with. Whether or not you agree with this is irrelevant. It is used to ensure that we build the proper support system around us. I recently saw a change to this quote attributed to Bernie Seigel, an expert in cancer treatment and holistic medicine. He changes the quote to say we are the average of the 4 people we spend the most time with, and his reasoning is that the number one person we spend the most time with is ourselves (In the spirit of full transparency, I did find this on Instagram, so it might not actually be his quote. However, I still totally agree with the statement regardless of its origins.).

I completely agree with this statement, and that is why before we work on our support cast, we need to improve our relationship with ourselves.

With the first habit, we learned that the people we interact with can either fill up or drain or proverbial cups. But we can also do this to ourselves. We are often more critical of ourselves than we are of others. We spend hours dwelling on something we should or should not have said. We keep ourselves up at night worrying about things that may or may not happen and the way people may or may not think of us. We learned that doing this adds additional stress which keeps us in a sympathetic state. As such, the additional stress does not allow us to properly recover.

In being overly critical of ourselves, we once again keep ourselves in that sympathetic state. We commit to a goal, but we expect it to go perfectly and never hit any roadblocks. That is a very unrealistic expectation of progress. A graph of real progress is not a straight line from zero to our goals. Instead, it is a curve with some loops, and it certainly includes some steps backwards. It sometimes even stops being graphed completely because we get sidetracked and have to come back to it another time.

Life is not all or nothing. We are often so quick to forgive others, but we forget that we are also human and will undoubtedly make mistakes. We sometimes think that having one cookie might ruin all of our goals, and then we convince ourselves to eat all of them plus an entire pizza because the day is already ruined. This all or nothing mentality is dangerous. We talked about it in the very first section of the book. As soon as we enter this mentality, we set ourselves up for failure. Putting food items on a no eat or forbidden list creates a strong desire for us to eat them. Instead of the all or nothing mentality, we can look at our choices on a continuum from not so healthy to healthy. We then strive to always be toward the healthy side of the continuum, but we understand that sliding toward the not so healthy side is not going to ruin our goals. It merely means that we are human. Sweet treats and processed foods are literally designed to make us crave them, and then consume as much of them as possible when we do. They are designed with sugar and fat levels that are not found in nature and are hyper palatable. Food companies literally hijack our taste buds and our minds. We will learn some tricks to set us up for success later within this habit. However, for now, we must be able to forgive ourselves.

Nobody is perfect. I definitely am not. I will tell you right now that anything my wife bakes is my weakness. Does that mean I am not going to enjoy the things she bakes? Of course, I will. Do I often feel guilty because it is not necessarily the healthiest option out there? Definitely. But then I remember what I would tell anyone that I am working with, "It happened, we can't change it, but there will be plenty more opportunities to be successful." It is paramount we remember to control only the things within our control. We can never control the past. But we always have control of right now.

Each day, each meal, each decision we make is an opportunity to reach our goals. If we happen to make a less than ideal choice, that is okay. We will have plenty more later. If we slide away from the healthiest options on the continuum, that is okay. We must simply accept it, and then we can work to slide back to health at the next opportunity. We are all continuously learning. If each day we work to try and be just a little bit better and get a little bit closer to our goals, we will be in a great place to reach our goals. Progress, no matter how big, is still progress. Be kind to yourself, love yourself, and remind yourself that you are human. Much like children, we need love and support to help us learn to make choices that align with our goals.

Unlike children, we can provide the calming voice of reason to ourselves. We can also define the person we want to be. Once we decide we are "a high caliber athlete who chooses to make healthy choices", or perhaps you are "a father who sets a healthy example for his children", or maybe you're a "positive person that helps others maintain their own health". It does not matter. Just decide who you are going to be and allow yourself to make the choices that person makes. Once we are in this mindset, success becomes much easier to obtain than when we self-degrade and belittle ourselves with negative comments and emotions. Self-talk is one of the most powerful tools we can utilize in helping us to reach our goals. It is critical to remember that our own actions can also fill up or drain our energy cups.

Nobody can do it alone, and now that we are in a better place with ourselves, we can build our support system. We are social creatures, and we perform best when we are cooperating and supporting each other. In fact, society as we know it today would never have come about if we never learned to cooperate. There is nothing more powerful than a group with a common goal pushing in the same direction. It is much more efficient than the individual approach. Small bands of people learned to trade with neighboring tribes, and the sheer number of items accessible to these tribes was able to grow along with the more tribes they were willing to trade with. As we learned to communicate better with one another, the capabilities of humans continued to grow, and our current realm of possibilities is nearly limitless. We have made tremendous economic, social, and technological growth due to cooperation. Cooperation is also one of the most common features within successful businesses.

Employees that feel safe to cooperate and are not fearful of the loss of their jobs are more likely to work harder and be more productive. I bet that if you were willing to look back on your most productive teams, in business, sport, or otherwise, those that saw the most success were those in which each member was able to play to their strengths while not feeling pressure or fear that the other members were only out for themselves.

Cooperation has even been shown to have a direct link to serotonin and oxytocin. These two chemicals are responsible for the feeling of well-being, pride, and respect when we accomplish something (serotonin) as well as the feeling of love or deep trust for those close to us (oxytocin). Simon Sinek calls these two the cooperation chemicals. They are called such because they increase when we can cooperate freely. Or just when we do nice things for other people. That feeling inside after you complete a selfless act, that is these two chemicals at work. When these two are depleted, we are more likely to commit selfish acts instead of selfless acts. So, in a situation where we do not feel supported or have the ability to cooperate, we are more likely to act in self-defense. Thus, a cycle of selfishness is created. Therefore, it is so critical we surround ourselves with individuals that will support us and allow us to support them. These positive social interactions have also been shown to help reduce the feeling of fatigue.

We all know these people. These are the people we immediately feel energized after speaking to. The people that we call when we are in a pinch because we know they have our back. We also know who these people are not. We feel drained after speaking to them. Or perhaps we dread speaking to them because we know that they either want something from us or will shoot down our ideas.

In addition to Sinek's work, Dr. Robert Sapolsky has another book called *Behave: The Biology of Humans at Our Best and Worst*. Within the book, he delves into the decision-making process and its influences varying from evolution millions of years ago to the milliseconds prior. He notes the positive effects of the hormones mentioned earlier. However, he also notes something else that happens in animal studies. Specifically, the hormone dopamine which commonly known as a "feel good hormone". However, recent findings suggest that it makes us act more in a way in which we already would. So, if we were already prone to violence, we would be more violent. If we were prone to kindness, we would be more kind. This shows how crucial it is that we choose our circle wisely. If we are afraid and uncertain within a circle, we will be more prone to act selfishly. However, in the right circle, we can act freely with the support of our circle, and our circle will cultivate the habits and routines in which these cooperation hormones truly have us act in cooperation. In fact, perfect examples are the best alpha males (those that remain in their position the longest) in the animal kingdom are not overly dominant. These hormones allow them to make choices that will allow them to stay in their position. What does that look like? Doing what is best for the group. This means that the alpha males are truly only alpha males when they are helping a group grow and flourish. It truly flips everything we thought we knew about alpha males doesn't it? We should all seek to be alphas in this regard. Hopefully, the first habit has allowed you to start noticing who these people are, and you have instinctually started spending more time with energizing people and less with draining people. But what is next?

Let us start with people in the house. If you are married, live with a significant other, or have a roommate, hopefully you have selected someone who you enjoy being with and you know has your back. Be clear with them with what you are planning on doing, what your goals are, and that you want their support. In a perfect world, they are willing to embark on this journey with you, and you can help each other as things progress and get more difficult. However, you may also need to have some difficult conversations about what you need from them other than support. For example, if you know sweets are something you cannot resist (this is how I am too), perhaps a house rule is created that sweets will not be kept in the house. This makes getting a sweet treat more difficult, but it also makes it special as you will need to leave the house to get your sweet fix (hello date night. It is a win-win). Or maybe there is a designated cabinet in the kitchen where the food you want to eat less of are kept. If you have the discipline to stay away from that cabinet, your partner can keep the things he or she wants around, and you never have to see or eat them.

Your situation is unique, so you may need to brainstorm with your coach or accountability buddy on exactly what you need. You are also free to tweak it as time goes on. Each situation will dictate what you need at that moment. The bottom line is that the best way to support someone is being clear with what each other's goals and expectations are, why they are what they are, and exactly what you need from each other to be successful. A good partner is going to support and understand you, and they will work to give you exactly what is needed. Be sure to be very clear on what you need and expect from them. It is much easier to meet expectations when they are clearly explained and out in the open.

We have now handled 2 of the 5 people you are closest to. You are kind and supporting of yourself, and you have the support of whomever you live with. Now it is time to build the rest of your supporting cast. The remaining 3 (or more, but try to keep it relatively small) can be anybody. This could even be a great reason to reach out to an old friend you have lost touch with. Or it might be a reason to reach out to somebody you might not be close with or know at all, but they embody the person you want to be. The who is not all that important. What they do is the most important. These people make you a better person. They push you to be and do your best in every situation, and they hold you accountable. They support your goals and find ways to accommodate your needs at any opportunlty. Pul simply, they fill your cup. You may start noticing your habits become a little bit easier. You start performing at work a little bit better. All your relationships are allowed to grow and flourish. Maybe you just feel better overall. Having a supporting cast of people we know, trust, and love can make a huge impact in every area of our lives. If these people are not in your life already, it might be time to re-evaluate your circle. I am not saying we need to cut people out of our lives completely, but most of our time should be spent with people that have our best interests in mind and want to help us be successful. To help you find these types people, there are 3 questions you can ask: 1) Are you committed to excellence? 2) Do you care about me? 3) Can I trust you? These questions were introduced to the Army West Point Football team when head coach Jeff Monken took over, and they are questions that have guided many of us when building our circle of trust.

It is also important that you find time to be with people in real life. Social media is a tremendous tool to be able to interact from a distance. However, it is no substitute for positive human interaction. Relationships are built face to face. We must allow ourselves to be vulnerable and be with people in the moment.

It might even be a good idea to begin to prune your social media feeds so that they are only bringing you information that is positive or relevant to your goals. Social media is often filled with negativity designed to bring negative emotions because that's how websites get more hits. While we should aim to spend less time on social media, we should work to make the time we do spend beneficial to us. This way it does not add any additional strain or stress to our lives, but instead helps to fill our cups. Take control of your feed and design it to be helpful. Otherwise, it can begin to be unhelpful at a very rapid pace.

One last note on therapy. I am a firm supporter of seeking help. I utilize a therapist, and it provides profound insights into myself that would have taken me a significantly long time, or I may never have even come across. There is nothing wrong with seeking help. A good therapist is someone you want in your circle. They can provide valuable insight, help you learn about yourself, and help you heal from trauma. Let us end the stigma surrounding therapy. We only get one brain, and we need to do everything we can to keep it healthy and running at its highest potential. We are also learning that the foods we eat can positively or negatively impact our psychological health. Exercise (or a lack thereof) can also play a large role in our psychological well-being. This is very exciting, and as you go through the habits throughout the book, you may recognize a shift in your psychological health. This is not to say that you should put off seeing a professional. A good one will likely be very aware of these findings and encourage your journey towards health.

We will dive deeper into how nutrition and exercise can help psychologically a bit later. For now, know that therapy is a tremendous tool to keep the brain healthy and help keep the balance of the psychology pillar. If you feel depressed, overwhelmed, stressed, unbalanced, out of whack, or something else you just cannot put your finger on, try working with a therapist to get to the bottom of it. We cannot do it all on our own. There is no need to try. Just like we want a coach to help us with our health goals, we want a good coach to help us keep our brains healthy. I will say that I tend to lean toward the body being able to balance itself out If glven the tools it needs. So, I would caution you to be wary of any practitioner in any field who merely prescribes something and advises you to come back multiple times instead of working to get to the deeper source of the problem. This individual likely just wants your money. We want practitioners that give us homework, that help us grow, and try to get to the root of our problems. This is not to say that medication does not have its merits and is not able to help many people. I have many friends who have seen the benefit, and I am so glad they were able to find something to help balance them. Because that is what it is all about right? Finding the solution that works best for us as an individual. I just want to help you find someone that is best suited to help you get what you need. You deserve that.

Even if you do not choose to see a therapist, it can be beneficial to talk things over with a trusted friend.

Always remember that you matter, you are relevant, and you are important. If you have thoughts of harming yourself or others, please call 1-800-273-8255.

Build Your Supporting Cast

Now that we have an idea of why it is important to build a strong supporting cast, we can get into how to implement the habit. The trick is to find what works best for you. We are all highly individual. I cannot tell you what is going to be best in your situation. That is something you must find on your own. A coach can help brainstorm ideas, but the execution falls on you. Use the notes section to brainstorm and track how different strategies work for you, and then work with your coach or accountability partner to really dial in what your best practice might be. Do not forget to continue the previous habits because they all work together. Focus on this habit for the next 4 weeks. Take more time if you need. Remember, we truly want this to become part of our lives.

- Take it Slow - Pick a person you want to add to your supporting cast. Ask them if they would like to be a part of your support system. Let them know what your goals are, and why you picked them. Try to come up with ideas either together or on your own of what they can specifically do to help you with your goals.

- A Little More Challenging - Pick 5 People you want to add to your supporting cast. The same rules apply as above.

- Ready for a Challenge - Pick 5 people you want to add to your supporting cast, but also make your goals public. This allows you to be held accountable in every situation. Tell your family, friends, and coworkers. Be specific with them on what they can do to help you accomplish their goals. See if any of them would like to join you.

Notes

General notes about the habit:

How are you planning on implementing this habit?

How ready, willing, and able are you to implement your strategy? (for a reminder on how to use this activity, see page 28)

What are some potential roadblocks you may face?

What are some strategies you can use prepare for these roadblocks?

What have you noticed about how you feel, think, or act after implementing this habit?

Which Pillars do you feel that this habit impacts? Why?

Any questions, comments, or concerns to bring up with your coach?

References

Berardi, J., & Andrews, R. (2010). *The essentials of sport and exercise nutrition*. Precision Nutrition.

Bubbs, M. (2019). *Peak: The new science of athletic performance that is revolutionizing sports* Chelsea Green Publishing.

Connolly, F., & White, P. (2017). *Game changer* Simon and Schuster

Coyle, D. (2018). *The culture code: The secrets of highly successful groups* Bantam.

Crockett, M. J., Clark, L., Lieberman, M. D., Tabibnia, G., & Robbins, T. W. (2010). Impulsive choice and altruistic punishment are correlated and increase in tandem with serotonin depletion. *Emotion, 10*(6), 855.

Dölen, G., Darvishzadeh, A., Huang, K. W., & Malenka, R. C. (2013). Social reward requires coordinated activity of nucleus accumbens oxytocin and serotonin. *Nature, 501*(7466), 179.

Harari, Y. N. (2014). *Sapiens: A brief history of humankind* Random House.

https://www.instagram.com/p/B6fmAOyJWYq/

Sapolsky, R. M. (2017). *Behave: The biology of humans at our best and worst* Penguin.

Sinek, S. (2014). *Leaders eat last: Why some teams pull together and others do not* Penguin.

Section III: The Food

Your mindset is in the right place, your sleep is on point, and your support system has been built. Now we can get to what you most likely came here for. You might already be feeling better or seeing results. You are absolutely nailing it! Keep it up!

Food can be confusing. There are numerous "superfoods" and other "health" foods out there. So many diets, and a million people saying contradicting things about certain foods. This section should hopefully shed some light on this confusing topic. Within you will find a guide on how to create portion sizes. Keep this in mind as you read through each habit.

The following page has an image to help you start building your meals, but we will dive deeper throughout this section. Each individual section will have a reminder at the end of the chapter, and this same image will appear at the end of the section. Remember, this is just a suggestion of where to start. Your actual needs might be different.

PORTION CONTROL GUIDE

FORGET CALORIE COUNTING. TRY THIS METHOD INSTEAD.

Most people think controlling portions means counting calories, but we think there's a better way.
Try our (much easier) Hand Measure system instead.

YOUR HAND IS ALL YOU NEED

Your hand is proportionate to your body, its size never changes, and it's always with you, making
it the perfect tool for measuring food and nutrients - minimal counting required.

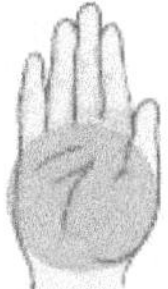

A serving of
protein =
1 PALM

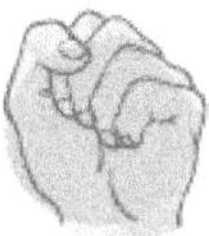

A serving of
vegetables =
1 FIST

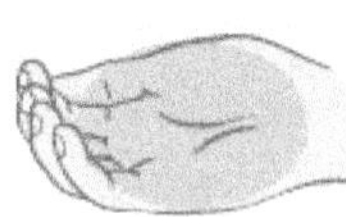

A serving of
carbs =
1 CUPPED HAND

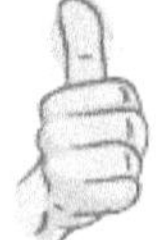

A serving of
fats =
1 THUMB

HERE'S HOW TO USE THIS METHOD TO BUILD A PLATE

STEP 1 → **STEP 2** → **STEP 3** → **STEP 4**

PROTEIN
Meat, fish, eggs, cottage cheese, and Greek yogurt

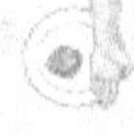
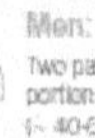

Women:
One palm-sized portion
(~ 20-30 g protein)

Men:
Two palm-sized portions
(~ 40-60 g protein)

VEGETABLES
Broccoli, spinach, salad, carrots, etc.

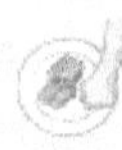
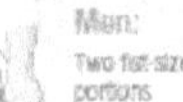

Women:
One fist-sized portion

Men:
Two fist-sized portions

CARBOHYDRATES
Grains, starches, beans, and fruits

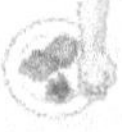
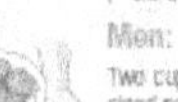
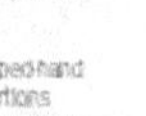

Women:
One cupped-hand sized portion
(~ 20-30 g carbs)

Men:
Two cupped-hand sized portions
(~ 40-60 g carbs)

FATS
Oils, butters, nut butters, nuts, and seeds

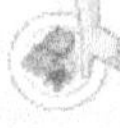

Women:
One thumb-sized portion
(~ 7-12 g fat)

Men:
Two thumb-sized portions
(~ 15-25 g fat)

Men eating 3-4 meals as outlined would get around 2,300 - 3,000 calories each day.
Women eating 3-4 meals as outlined would get around 1,200 - 1,500 calories each day.

NOW, CUSTOMIZE THE PLAN FOR YOU

Active **men** do best with 6-8 servings of each food group per day (~2,300-3,000 kcal).
Active **women** do best with 4-6 servings of each food group per day (~1,500 - 2,100 kcal).
From there, adjust the number of portions to meet your personal needs and goals.

IF YOU NEED MORE FOOD BECAUSE YOU...

- Are larger in stature
- Aren't getting muscle-gain results
- Eat less frequently throughout the day
- Are very active
- Are trying to gain muscle
- Aren't feeling satisfied at meals

...THEN START BY ADDING...

Men: 1 cupped handful of carbs and/or 1 thumb of fat to a few meals each day.
Women: 1/2 cupped handful of carbs and/or 1/2 thumb of fat to a few meals each day.

IF YOU NEED LESS FOOD BECAUSE YOU...

- Are smaller in stature
- Aren't getting weight-loss results
- Eat more frequently throughout the day
- Are not very active
- Are trying to lose weight
- Are feeling too full at meals

...THEN START BY REMOVING...

Men: 1 cupped handful of carbs and/or 1 thumb of fat from a few meals each day.
Women: 1/2 cupped handful of carbs and/or 1/2 thumb of fat from a few meals each day.

This system is easier than counting calories and nearly as accurate. Just like with counting, though, pay attention to results and adjust as needed.

For the full article explaining this infographic:
https://www.precisionnutrition.com/calorie-control-guide

 **Precision**Nutrition

Habit 5: Water

Quite frankly, water is the only liquid we need to be drinking (although with a 6-month-old, I am currently fueled by large amounts of coffee). But why is water so important? Well here are some numbers to consider: bone is about 22% water, adipose (fat) tissue is about 25% water, muscle and brain tissue are about 75% water, blood is about 83% water, and eyes are about 95% water. Two-thirds of our bodies are made up of water. Water plays a critical role in our hydration, detoxification, and electrolyte balance. It lubricates, regulates our temperature, and transports nutrients to and from our cells. Bottom line: we need water to be healthy. Men should shoot for 3.7 Liters, and women should shoot for 2.7 Liters each day. Activity levels, body size, and electrolyte balance will ultimately dictate whether we need more, or less. However, these are good numbers to begin to aim for.

Even more interesting is that we have not learned all there is to know about water yet. A new fourth phase of water has recently been discovered, and the implications on science and our health is still being discovered. This fourth phase, called EZ water, is a liquid crystalline. It is not quite liquid, but not quite a solid either. It envelopes every single macromolecule within our cells. It even has implications for the body being able to heal itself when properly hydrated.

Without adequate levels of hydration, we will be unable to perform physically or cognitively. Physical performance begins to decline with just 2% lost water weight, and cognitive performance begins to decline with 5%. To make matters worse, most of us are under consuming water. Our days are filled with sugar-filled drinks which give us a small boost short term, and then lead to a crash not long after. We then quickly go for another boost, and this continues throughout the day. This can lead to some serious health implications.

Water contributing to healing and ultimately fueling our goals is not really news. However, somewhere along the line with the plethora of beverage choices, we seemed to have forgotten this critical piece of our health. The discovery of EZ water does create somewhat of a buzz, but water just is not interesting. It is plain, it is boring, and sometimes we just need more than water. But, in truth, water is the only liquid we need despite what our taste buds might tell us.

We have a large selection of beverages to choose from. Most of these do more damage than they help us. With the discussion around ultra-processed foods swirling in the media, one might think that these foods are the largest contributor to sugar in our diets. It is actually sugar sweetened beverages that is the biggest contributor to sugar in our diets. And individuals who consume large amounts of sugar, have the highest rates of obesity, heart disease, diabetes, and cancer. We know soda is a large factor in sugary beverage consumption. But, sports drinks, coffee drinks, and fruit juices are also 3 of the biggest contributors to our added sugar problem.

It is important that we discuss how sugar impacts our bodies. When we consume sugar, our bodies respond by producing insulin. In small quantities, this is not an issue as we need this for our tissues to take glucose within the cells. However, when we ingest too much, our cells become saturated. At this point we can no longer hold any additional glucose within our cells. Our bodies create more insulin to tell our cells we need to get the glucose out of our blood stream. This excess glucose will eventually be converted into adipose tissue to be used later when the body needs it. However, when we continue to ingest sugar, we begin to become resistant to insulin, and we store more and more glucose as adipose. This leads into Insulin resistance, metabolic disease, and Type 2 Diabetes in conjunction with the diseases that these all have links to such as cardiovascular disease, obesity, and Alzheimer's (starting to more frequently be called type 3 diabetes due to its link to insulin resistance and inflammation). This is an ultra-simplified explanation of the impact sugar has within our bodies. This also happens in conjunction with a multitude of other metabolic functions within our bodies. For a more detailed explanation, check out the references or further reading sections.

These issues become exacerbated by the fact that ultra-processed foods are created in a manner that makes us want more. If this all occurs along with a high stress environment, lack of exercise, and poor sleep, we get what James LaValle, author of *Cracking the Metabolic Code,* calls the Downward Spiral of Health. All these things contribute to an environment within our bodies resulting in a continued state of inflammation and disease which result in chronic health issues.

Despite what advertisers might want us to believe, most of us do not need a sports drink after a workout. They are made specifically for athletes participating in long events. Even then, a more diluted solution than what typically comes in a bottle is needed as opposed to the high sugar content of what we can pick up on the shelves at the grocery store. Coffee has some tremendous health benefits. It contains antioxidants and can give you an energy boost if you need it. The issue with coffee comes forward when we add sugar. Flavors, syrups, whipped cream, and just plain sugar all have similar metabolic effects when we consume them. Most commercially available drinks also come loaded with all these things. And then we have fruit juices. These are often labeled as healthy, but they affect us the same as sodas and other drinks with sugars added. Even fruit juices with no added sugars bring forward the same responses within our bodies. The reason for this is that we do not get any of the fiber or other nutrients when we consume these juices. Plus, the amount required to create them is significantly higher than if we simply choose to eat the fruit instead.

To counter this, many companies and people are switching to artificial sweeteners. No Calories, so it is a healthy alternative. Simple solution, right? Unfortunately, this is not the case, artificial sweeteners have a similar metabolic response to sugar. In fact, they have been shown to change our gut microbiome, and have been shown to make us consume more due to the alteration in the microbiome. To make matters worse, the body thinks it is going to get

X number of Calories from these sweeteners, but it does not get those Calories. This also creates the urge to consume more.

One potential alternative to sugar and artificial sweeteners are sugar alcohols. They have a low insulin response and can even help our beneficial gut bacteria. Some people do experience bloating, gas, and discomfort. If this is the case for you, you are not alone because it is for me too. If so, it may be best to avoid sugar alcohols as well. It is possible that this is alleviated once a healthy balance is restored to our gut microbiome, so it may be beneficial to retry later if you do experience these symptoms.

We talked about alcohol within our habit on sleep. It is also important we discuss it here. There is some research to suggest that moderate (roughly one or two drinks a day) consumption of alcohol could lead to increased longevity. This is more specifically the case with wine which does include polyphenols and antioxidants. As consumption increases, longevity and health have been shown to decrease. Consuming more than 2 alcoholic beverages in a single sitting has been linked to decreased fat burning a couple of hours following the consumption. Many beers contain extra Calories along with a large amount of carbohydrates, and many cocktails have added sugar. Since the body already must work to detoxify the alcohol from our systems, added sugar may not be in our best interest. Alcohol also creates cravings for more unhealthy food options when consumed in excess. We already understand the impact alcohol has on sleep, so we do not need to dive into that more here. For a refresher, feel free to jump back into the sleep habit. It is important to note the negative impact alcohol has outside of sleep. Alcohol does not allow us to fully recover from exercise since it inhibits cellular repair. It reduces testosterone and other growth producing hormones and can prevent memories being moved into long term storage thanks to its impact on sleep. Serotonin is also decreased leading to an increased likelihood of depression. Alertness and reaction time are also negatively impacted by alcohol, and this is not just the case right after consumption. These are all effects that last well into the days following a night out of drinking.

This information is by no means an attempt to dissuade you from consuming alcohol. I still partake in the occasional alcoholic drink (sometimes too frequently). This information is an attempt to educate you on the impacts the things you consume can have on your goals and your health. You are capable of making your own decisions, and I encourage you to do so. If you are looking to consume alcohol, just remember moderation. We are also better off sticking with wine and hard alcohol if we are looking to reduce the number of sugars and additives.

When looking for teas and coffees, it is best to go with organic and fair-trade certified products. This ensures workers and farmers are getting a fair price for their products, and that the ingredients used are not going to carry any added toxins. We will talk more about organic products when we discuss vegetables in detail. However, for now it is important to remember that we get what we pay for. To ensure that what we consume is doing more good than harm, we should try to always get the highest quality products when possible.

Drink water. This habit really boils down to that statement. It is simple in theory, but sometimes difficult in execution. There are some ways we can make water a little more interesting. Infused water is one trick. It gives it some flavor but does not take away from the benefits of water. Filter your water. There are even some stainless-steel bottles that come with filters. Reverse osmosis filters are the gold standard, but there are many others that can do a good job if you are not ready to commit to a reverse osmosis filter. The chemical flavor we are so accustomed to comes from additives within the purification process. This process is necessary because current agricultural practices leak toxins and pesticides into water sources and damage local ecosystems. Well water and ice melts are great sources of water if possible. However, if it is coming from an area near a conventional farm, it may be significantly worse.

How do we know if we have enough water? Our pee is a great indicator of our hydration level. Clear is very hydrated, and a light lemonade color is well hydrated. The darker our pee gets, the less hydrated we are. If your pee is brown, begin to drink water immediately. If you find blood in your urine, seek medical attention.

When in doubt, drink water. Try adding a glass first thing in the morning. We are often dehydrated upon waking, and when coffee is the first thing we go for, we put ourselves at a greater disadvantage. Avoid bottled water as this creates a large environmental strain. Any drink that is adding additional Calories to our diets is typically a no-go. Also, we want to look out for waters containing flavoring, coloring, or sweeteners. However, here are some guidelines to help you along the way. Try to get water in its most pure form. Filters are our friend when it comes to water consumption. The purer we can get our water, the better. Teas, especially green tea, and coffee are okay. Try not to overdo it on the coffee and try to brew teas at home. When purchasing from a vendor, be careful about added sugars. Sugars manage to sneak their way into most consumer goods. Instead of juice, try vegetable and fruit smoothies, but do not add extra juice to it. Try to stick with low glycemic fruits such as berries.

Water

Now that we have an idea of why it is important to get plenty of water, we can get into how to implement the habit. The trick is to find what works best for you. We are all highly individual. I cannot tell you what is going to be best in your situation. That is something you must find on your own. A coach can help brainstorm ideas, but the execution falls on you. Use the notes section to brainstorm and track how different strategies work for you, and then work with your coach or accountability partner to really dial in what your best practice might be. Do not forget to continue the previous habits because they all work together. Focus on this habit for the next 4 weeks. Take more time if you need. Remember, we truly want this to become part of our lives.

- Take it Slow - Simply add an extra glass of water to your daily routine. A great place for this is the first thing in the morning as we are typically dehydrated upon waking. We worsen our dehydration when coffee is the first thing we consume. Try infusing your water if you need a little flavor but try to work towards plain water.

- A Little More Challenging - Add 2-3 additional glasses of water each day. Begin to track your liquid consumption. Notice if you have a lot of sugary drinks. Use the notes section to start developing a plan to increase water consumption. Drink alcohol in moderation.

- Ready for a Challenge - Only drink water. You can have some coffee or tea but be careful with what you (or someone else) add to it. Plain is best. Start to notice and track how you feel as you consume more water. If you choose to drink alcohol, do so responsibly and in moderation. Try to stick with wine or hard alcohol

Notes

General notes about the habit:

How are you planning on implementing this habit?

How ready, willing, and able are you to implement your strategy? (for a reminder on how to use this activity, see page 28)

What are some potential roadblocks you may face?

What are some strategies you can use prepare for these roadblocks?

What have you noticed about how you feel, think, or act after implementing this habit?

Which Pillars do you feel that this habit impacts? Why?

Any questions, comments, or concerns to bring up with your coach?

References

Bae, J., Park, J., Im, S., & Song, D. (2014). Coffee and health. *Integrative Medicine Research, 3*(4), 189-191.

Berardi, J., & Andrews, R. (2010). *The essentials of sport and exercise nutrition.* Precision Nutrition.

Bubbs, M. (2019). *Peak: The new science of athletic performance that is revolutionizing sports* Chelsea Green Publishing.

Connolly, F., & White, P. (2017). *Game changer* Simon and Schuster.

Hyman, M. (2018). *Food: What the heck should I eat?* Hachette UK.

Hyman, M. (2020). *Food Fix: How to Save Our Health, Our Economy, Our Communities, and Our Planet -- One Bite at a Time.* Little, Brown Spark

LaValle, J. B., & Yale, S. L. (2004). *Cracking the metabolic code: The nine keys to peak health* Basic Health Publications, Inc.

Learney, P. (2014). *N1 nutritional programming: the fundamentals of nutritional programming.* ACA.

Pollack, G. H. (2013a). The fourth phase of water. *Ebner & Sons Publishers, Seattle, Washington,*

Pollack, G. H. (2013b). The fourth phase of water: Beyond solid. *Liquid, and Vapor,*

Suez, J., Korem, T., Zeevi, D., Zilberman-Schapira, G., Thaiss, C. A., Maza, O., Weinberger, A. (2014). Artificial sweeteners induce glucose intolerance by altering the gut microbiota. *Nature, 514*(7521), 181.

Swithers, S. E. (2013). Artificial sweeteners produce the counterintuitive effect of inducing metabolic derangements. *Trends in Endocrinology & Metabolism, 24*(9), 431-441.

Verstegen, M., & Williams, P. (2014). *Every day is game day: Train like the pros with a no-holds-barred exercise and nutrition plan for peak performance* Penguin.

Habit 6: Protein

Let us get this out of the way early. I personally believe that meat is the best source of protein for us. It contains a host of vitamins and minerals, and when sourced properly, meat is the best way for us to ensure we are getting enough protein. It is also essential to heal our soil and reverse the effects of climate change. For this habit, I am going to suggest you do consume quality meat. But it will not be just meat, there will also be guidelines for poultry, eggs, milk/dairy, and seafood. We evolved eating meat, and I spoke earlier on how our digestive tracts are suited for eating a variety of foods and not just plants or meats. The issue is much of the protein sources on the market simply are not sourced properly. We will go over what we should be looking for when we are picking our protein sources. We will also dive into why we probably need to be avoiding things like plant based, meat-like food. If you are a vegan, you probably hate me now. Do not worry, we are going to discuss ways to ensure you are getting enough quality proteins, and how to allow the habits of this chapter to work for your situation. It is just much more difficult. The reason is that the sources of proteins that are derived solely from plants lack several essential amino acids. What is an essential amino acid you might be thinking? Well, let us get into some of the science of protein.

Proteins are amino acids that are joined by peptide bonds. We begin to break them down as we are chewing, and then they go through the digestive pathway we discussed earlier. The goal of digestion is to break the proteins down into the smallest possible parts. So, the more we can do in our mouths, the easier time our bodies will have absorbing the proteins and other nutrients. Exactly where these amino acids go, and what they do for our bodies depends on what we need at the time. For the most part, about 20% will be used by the liver for protein synthesis, about 60% will be catabolized (broken down) by the liver, and about 20% will go into circulation. Our bodies have a pool of amino acids which it uses to recover our muscles and connective tissue after a tough workout, synthesize neurotransmitters, enzymes, and immune system chemicals. To do all of these things the amino acid pool needs to be filled with the necessary amino acids. When this is not the case, we begin to see the body breakdown other materials for the more essential functions.

As you can see, there are many functions that amino acids, and subsequently protein, are responsible. It is critical we ensure that our bodies are getting enough through our diets. Our bodies can make 12 amino acids on its own. These are called the non-essential amino acids. There are 8 essential amino acids that we must get from the food we eat. In some situations, the body will need extra amino acids. These are called conditionally essential amino acids, and there are 8 of them. These help when we are young and growing, when we need to recover from a difficult workout, or when we need to recover from an injury or illness. We can make them, but it is not always efficient.

How much we need also depends on a few factors. Men are larger and typically need a little more than women, active individuals will need a little more, and those recovering from injury and illness will also benefit from some extra amino acids within the pool. Protein helps to keep us full longer, so those looking to lose weight may benefit from having more protein in the diet as well. If you like numbers, 0.8 grams per kilogram (g/kg) of bodyweight per day is probably about as low as you want to go. If you are an elite level athlete, you can take it as high as about 2.2 g/kg of bodyweight per day. If you are a recreational athlete, or just an active person, you probably want to be somewhere in the middle. 20-30 grams 3-4 times a day is a great place to start. If you are more of a visual person, open your hand with your palm facing you. Look at your palm, and that is about what we want our protein size to be. 1-2 palm-sized 3-4 times per day will likely get us within the same ballpark, and since our palms are relative to our body size, it is a lot easier than counting grams per kilogram. As Dr. Mark Hyman, functional medicine practitioner and author, points out in his book *Food: What the Heck Should I Eat*, meat should be thought of more as a condiment than the main portion of our meals. We want our plates to be mostly colorful vegetables along with smaller amounts of grains, meats, and fats. We also want our meat to be of the highest quality to ensure we are not doing more damage to our bodies than we are good.

We now know how much but let us get into what types we should be eating.

Red meat often gets a bad rap. This is partly because of the myth that saturated fats are going to kill us. However, the link between saturated fat and heart disease has been disproven. Not to mention, quality meats contain more than just saturated fats. Quality sourced meats contain more omega-3 fats than omega-6 fats. We will discuss fats in more detail within the next habit. However, for now we can focus on the idea that fat is not bad for us, omega-3's are anti-inflammatory, and omega-6's are pro-inflammatory. The closer we can get the ratio of omega-6 to omega-3 to 2:1, the better off we will be.

So, why does meat today get such a bad rap? The answer is in how meat today is produced. Most of our meat comes from feedlot cows, and this also applies to chickens, pigs, and un-sustainably farmed fish. These animals are given harsh and unsanitary conditions, high stress environments, and given antibiotics to keep them fat as well as just healthy enough to stay alive until it is time to go to slaughter. Antibiotics are sold in higher qualities for farmed animals than for people. We learned earlier that stress can do some serious damage if we stay in a sympathetic state and not be allowed to get into a parasympathetic state. We get a slew of inflammatory hormones that cause damage to our bodies. If this is happening in the food we eat, don't you think we might see similar effects when we consume it? The fact of the matter is that what our food eats is very important when it comes to our health.

Antibiotics help keep the animals fat, but what else is legally allowed in the food of feedlot cows? Cows are typically fed mostly grains. Grains are known to increase fat and mass of the animals (it does the same in humans which we will discuss in the carbohydrate habit). Feather meal; recycled animal waste (poop, we are feeding these animals poop); food containing waste from rodents, insects, or birds (more poop); plastic; and some toxic chemicals. These animals are also often fed sugar, candy, and potato chips. Sometimes these things are still in the wrappers. I do not know about you, but none of that sounds like anything I would want to eat. Our bodies have enough to worry about without the added strain of detoxifying more stress hormones from our food. Not only are these factory farms contributing to our disease, but they also create a heavy weight on our environment.

Let us imagine a not so dystopian future, as Yuval Harari does in his book *Homo Deus a Brief History of Tomorrow*. Imagine that AI is now the predominant leader of society, and they have learned from our example. Now, we are being exploited and treated the same way we treat many animals – held in unsanitary, cluttered conditions where we are not allowed to fully live our lives. The needs of AI outweigh our own much like our needs seem to outweigh that of animals today. Hardly seems like an ideal situation to me.

Granted this is an exaggeration and a very slippery slope, and some things are already being done to improve the treatment of these animals as well as the food system in general. However, we must understand that animals and our environment are not simply things to be exploited by us. We must learn to properly treat these animals. Not only for their well-being, but also because it gives us more healthy options for consumption. We should be thankful for their sacrifice that allows us to live. One day, we will become the ground on which these animals feed. A wise lion once called it the circle of life.

So, where should our meat come from? Grass-fed grass-finished meat is the ideal meat we should be consuming. It has less strain on the environment, and the animals are allowed the courtesy of living the way nature intended. Grass-fed meat is significantly better for us than commercially farmed meat, that is nearly an entirely different food. When animals are allowed to graze and forage, they absorb more nutrients from the ground. They are healthier, and do not need antibiotics to keep them alive or fatten them up. As they graze and forage, these animals also provide nutrients to the soil. This is a big deal as our soil has started to decrease the amount of nutrients within it thanks to the way we currently farm. Grass-fed meats also contain more omega-3's than their grain fed counterparts, are less likely to be contaminated with superbugs or bacteria and have higher levels of vitamins and minerals. These animals live happier, healthier lives, and are not filled with the stress hormones that can cause us damage.

These same principles apply to poultry and eggs, pork, and seafood. The closer we can get to their natural environment and diet, the more nutritious they will be for us. They are also less likely to carry diseases which can be transmitted to us. When choosing our protein sources, organically fed animals within their natural habitat (free-range, grass-fed, pastured, foraging, wild caught) is what we should be looking for. In the instance of seafood, smaller is better. Larger fish tend to have higher instances of mercury which can cause significant damage to our bodies. Any fish larger than a normal plate is probably too large and is best if avoided.

Protein sourced in these methods is typically more expensive. However, the typical western diet consists of far too much anyway. In consuming less, but higher quality protein sources, you will likely see the cost balance out long term. Not to mention, it is an investment towards your own health. We can either pay for it now or pay more over the long term. As we start to demand more quality sources of food in general, it forces companies to re-evaluate their methods and products, and in an ideal situation will drive prices down creating a situation in which quality sourced foods simply becomes food. Until this time, we need to vote with our dollars and demand high quality food sources. There are even companies such as ButcherBox that will deliver high quality meat right to your door. This is something we use, and we absolutely love it. The meat tastes great, and we do not have to worry about the quality!

For you plant-based eaters, do not worry. I have not forgotten about you. Here are some things to consider: Make sure you are eating enough. Plant based foods tend to require you to eat more. Eat a large variety. As much variety as possible will ensure you are getting plenty of nutrients and keeping your amino acid pool filled. Avoid building your diet around cereals, grains, and other processed foods. Just like these things fatten up cattle, they have similar effects when we consume them. They are also much less nutritious than their whole food counterparts.

It may be necessary to supplement. We will talk supplements specifically toward the end of the book. But this is important for this population. Thus, we are going to talk about it a bit here. I mentioned earlier that it is challenging to meet your energy needs. This is especially true if you are an active person. It could be necessary to supplement with a plant-based protein powder. There are many out there, but the best I have found (there is some on my counter right now, so I am not just talking out of my rear end) is Momentous. It tastes great, contains all of the essential amino acids, and it is sourced from the highest quality ingredients. You may also be low in iron and some other vitamins and minerals. If you are not feeling 100%, and seem to be fatigued and lethargic, an iron supplement might be beneficial. However, to truly dial in your deficiencies, it would be a good idea to get blood work done and then work to fill in your gaps.

Avoid meat replica foods. Check the ingredients list out. It has a plethora of added stuff in there that we should not be consuming such as unhealthy oils and other additives that should not be consumed. If you are going to be plant-based, focus on whole foods. Everyone needs to be focusing on whole foods anyway. These imposter foods and much of the packaged goods out there are advertised as healthy, but that just is not the case.

Now we have the what and the how much. Just a quick recap though. 0.8 grams per kilogram (g/kg) of bodyweight per day is probably about as low as you want to go. If you are an elite level athlete, you can take it as high as about 2.2 g/kg of bodyweight per day. If you are a recreational athlete, or just an active person, you probably want to be somewhere in the middle. 20-30 grams 3-4 times a day is a great place to start. If you are more of a visual person, open up your hand with your palm facing you. Look at your palm, and that is about what we want our protein size to be. 1-2 palm-sized servings 3-4 times per day will likely get us within the same ballpark, and since our palms are relative to our body size, it is a lot easier than counting grams per kilogram. Remember, meat is more of a condiment than a main portion.

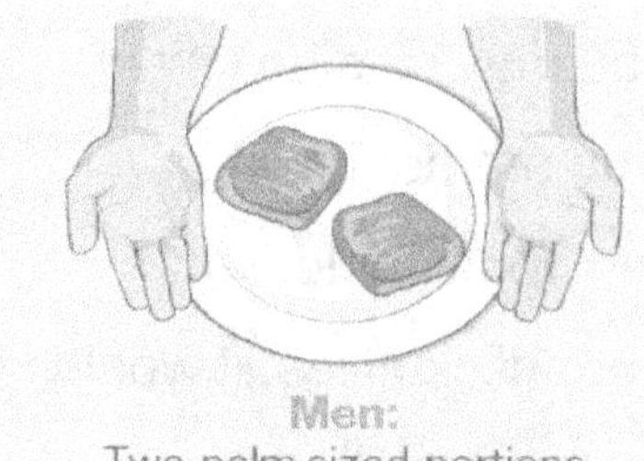

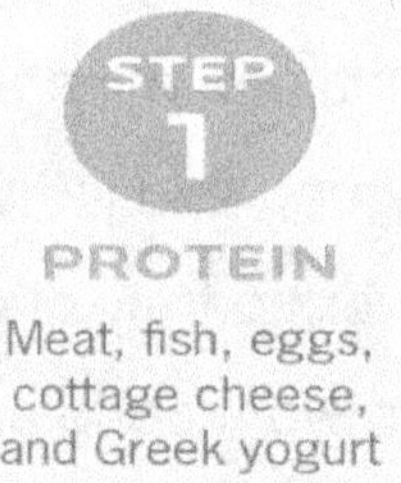

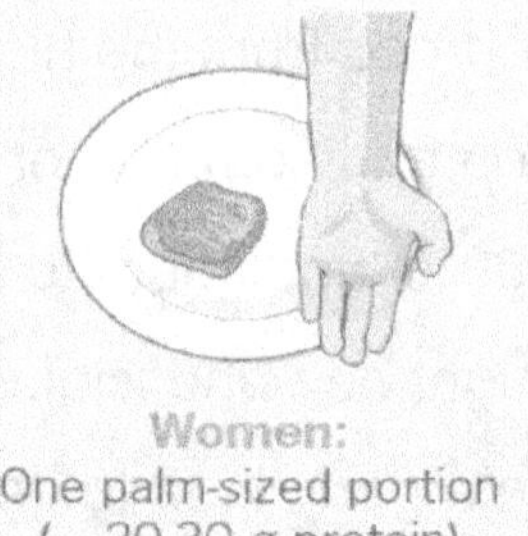

Protein

Now that we have an idea of why it is important to consume quality protein, we can get into how to implement the habit. The trick is to find what works best for you. We are all highly individual. I cannot tell you what is going to be best in your situation. That is something you must find on your own. A coach can help brainstorm ideas, but the execution falls on you. Use the notes section to brainstorm and track how different strategies work for you, and then work with your coach or accountability partner to really dial in what your best practice might be. Do not forget to continue the previous habits because they all work together. Focus on this habit for the next 4 weeks. Take more time if you need. Remember, we truly want this to become part of our lives.

- Take it Slow - Pick a single meal during the week, and replace your protein serving with a palm sized portion of quality sourced example from above. Use the notes section to notice the difference in taste, texture, and how you feel.

- A Little More Challenging - Pick 3-4 meals during the week and replace your protein servings with a palm sized portion of a quality sourced examples from above. Use the notes section to notice the difference in taste, texture, and how you feel.

- Ready for a Challenge - Replace all your protein servings with a palm sized portion of a quality sourced examples from above. Use the notes section to notice the difference in taste, texture, and how you feel.

Notes

General notes about the habit:

How are you planning on implementing this habit?

How ready, willing, and able are you to implement your strategy? (for a reminder on how to use this activity, see page 28)

What are some potential roadblocks you may face?

What are some strategies you can use prepare for these roadblocks?

What have you noticed about how you feel, think, or act after implementing this habit?

Which Pillars do you feel that this habit impacts? Why?

Any questions, comments, or concerns to bring up with your coach?

References

Berardi, J., & Andrews, R. (2010). *The essentials of sport and exercise nutrition.* Precision Nutrition.

Bubbs, M. (2019). *Peak: The new science of athletic performance that is revolutionizing sports* Chelsea Green Publishing.

Connolly, F., & White, P. (2017). *Game changer* Simon and Schuster.

Harari, Y. N. (2014). *Sapiens: A brief history of humankind* Random House.

Harari, Y. N. (2016). *Homo deus: A brief history of tomorrow* Random House.

https://www.precisionnutrition.com/calorie-control-guide-infographic

Hyman, M. (2018). *Food: What the heck should I eat?* Hachette UK.

Hyman, M. (2020). *Food Fix: How to Save Our Health, Our Economy, Our Communities, and Our Planet -- One Bite at a Time.* Little, Brown Spark

LaValle, J. B., & Yale, S. L. (2004). *Cracking the metabolic code: The nine keys to peak health* Basic Health Publications, Inc.

Learney, P. (2014). *N1 nutritional programming: The fundamentals of nutritional programming.* ACA

Taubes, G. (2007). *Good calories, bad calories* Anchor.

Verstegen, M., & Williams, P. (2014). *Every day is game day: Train like the pros with a no-holds-barred exercise and nutrition plan for peak performance* Penguin.

Habit 7: Carbohydrates

Carbohydrates are typically divided into monosaccharides, oligosaccharides, and polysaccharides. Basically, this is how many sugar molecules are linked together. That is right, carbohydrates are just sugar. The good news is that this does not make every carbohydrate out there unhealthy. I am sure you have heard that you want to stick with "complex" carbohydrates. Unfortunately, this is not the whole picture. We will get into what we should eat, and what we should avoid. For now, ditch the complex carb over simple carb rule. We do want slower-digesting carbohydrates such as fruits, whole grains, and some beans and legumes. As we eat carbohydrates, our bodies must work to break them down into their simplest form, glucose, so that the body can use them.

Let us start with a simple question. Are granola bars healthy? Nope. They are just glorified cookies. Grains are something we do not have to consume at all. Most grains in the United States contain glyphosate – a toxic substance found in pesticides we definitely want to avoid. There are other foods that are excellent sources of carbohydrates with much more added benefit.

The reason is that refined carbohydrates such as flour have a slightly different molecular makeup than sugar. We talked about what sugar does to insulin when we consume it in the water habit. In fact, sugar and grains have a similar glycemic index rating. This is the rating given to a food based on how much it raises our insulin. You may have heard that simply cutting Calories is the way to lose weight. This is only partially true. What we now know is that some Calories are can be better for gaining weight, and some are better for losing. Fats are great if we want to lose weight. If we want to gain weight, and increase our chances for cancer, diabetes, and even mental illness, refined carbohydrates are the way to go.

Knowing that refined carbohydrates are great at helping us gain weight and increase our chances of disease, here is an excerpt from *Food: What the Heck Should I Eat?* to truly paint a picture of how twisted our food system currently is:

> Grain-based foods are by far the number one source of calories in the American diet. Among adults, the number one source of calories is baked desserts, followed by yeast breads, and among adolescents and teenagers, the number two source of calories is pizza - in other words, flour and cheese. The grains that go into those foods - mainly wheat, corn, rice, and sorghum - are among the crops that receive billions in federal farm subsidies annually, so even our tax dollars are devoted to keeping grain-based foods like bread, pasta, rice, cereals, cookies, cake, pizza, oatmeal, and crackers on top. And it does not stop

there. Most of these federally subsidized crops are fed to livestock, which means that Americans are also getting grains indirectly, too, from all the grain-fed beef, chicken, and dairy we consume. The average American consumes 133 pounds of flour a year in their food (down from 146.8 pounds in 1995); that is more than a third of a pound per person per day, and some of us consume much more. And that does not include all the other grains and potatoes. We were never designed to handle this much starch. It is a toxic drug dose that leads to obesity, heart disease, type 2 diabetes, dementia, and even cancer.

This paints a grim picture. The current food system is literally setting us up for failure and disease. We do not even need to eat grains. There are no essential grains. We did not start consuming them regularly until we began farming it. Since our ancestors used to be able to move around and go where the food was, they were free to move wherever they pleased. and it could be argued that we became slaves to grains instead of the other way around due to farming.

To make the case for grains even worse, many of them contain gluten, and our bodies have no idea how to process gluten. Even if you do not have a diagnosis for Celiac's disease, most of us still have a negative response to gluten known as non-celiac gluten sensitivity. What this means is that most of us still have an inflammatory response when we consume gluten. We just do not feel it as someone with Celiac's disease would. Thus, we are still doing damage to our cells. It is just more of a slow burn. Companies are now making a killing selling "gluten-free" products. This is more bad news for us. Some of the replacements for gluten do just as much damage. These products are highly processed. A gluten-free cookie is still loaded with sugar, and a gluten-free waffle is still highly processed. If you are adding syrup to your gluten-free waffles, you are upping the sugar even more. The best gluten free products are whole foods.

Breakfast cereals, bagels, and oatmeal are all things we can do without. In starting our day with a high carbohydrate content, we spike our insulin and we crash before lunch time even comes around. We are hungrier soon after eating and instinctively reach for the next item that is going to spike our energy (often a soda, granola bar, or something along those lines). Oatmeal can be a good tool for those looking to gain weight if sourced properly but avoid instant and microwavable (we want to avoid microwaving food as a rule anyway) oatmeal. Save the oatmeal for your post workout or nighttime shake if you are looking to gain weight. We will get into how to shape our meals in the next section, but for now, just ditch the carbohydrates in the morning. You might notice your energy levels stay the same throughout the day.

Are some grains good for us? Yes. There are plenty of nutrients in whole grains. Unfortunately, this does not make whole grain bread and cereal good for us. For a product to be labeled as whole grain, the flour used to create the product simply needs to come from whole grains. Meaning they still get smashed into flour, and still create a high insulin response. Much of the nutrients are removed in this process.

In fact, very common high-carbohydrate foods started out as a quest to lower the male libido. Kellogg and Graham (you may recognize those names as some of the larger processed food companies) believed that the male sexual desire was at the root of all evil. So, they wanted to create foods that were bland and could reduce the impact of that sexual desire. Turns out, they may have been on to something as these types of foods have big implications for our hormones.

Now that you are super bummed out about grains, we can talk about the grains we can eat. Focus on the "weird" grains. Things like millet, buckwheat, amaranth, quinoa, and black rice. Some of these are often called "ancient grains". They are even better for us when they are sprouted grains. This happens when they are soaked. Did you know there are actually different colors of rice? There are, and the colorful variations have plenty of nutrients and antioxidants. If you are looking for a bread option, look for bread with whole kernels and seeds. Also make sure that there is no added sugar. Maybe even experiment with making your own from different types of flour like almond or coconut flour.

Starches do not fare much better. They also produce a high insulin response. Bad news for the mashed potato lovers out there. Does this mean you can never have mashed potatoes? Of course not. But each situation is different. One interesting fact about starches is that when cooked and then cooled, they become more resistant (resistant starches resist the digestive process) and are better for us since they feed the good bacteria in our guts. So, we might want to enjoy our potatoes and pasta (always homemade with quality ingredients, most pastas we buy in the store are highly processed and not very good for us) after we cool them. Remember that we want to go organic to maximize our nutrient content and reduce exposure to pesticides and other toxins.

Now for the easy part: fruits and vegetables. Eat them. Eat as many as you can and eat them as often as you can. Seriously, it is that easy. The more color and variety we can incorporate, the more nutrients and benefits we will get. This is especially true for vegetables. They help keep the bacteria in our guts happy, and we want them happy (they produce most of the serotonin in our bodies!). You might have heard that the fructose in fruits are bad for us. When we consume fructose, or high fructose corn syrup, this is the case. These things have been linked to weight gain, diabetes, and disease. But, when we consume fructose in its naturally occurring form from a whole fruit, I would say it is significantly better than the ultra-processed alternatives out there. The fiber from the fruit acts as a sort of buffer for fructose. I still suggest eating more vegetables than fruits. Maybe you need to start slowly and ween your body from the sugar. That is for you to decide.

If you know you are insulin resistant (if you do not know, but you have a little extra belly fat than you would like, you likely are. Do not worry that is where it affects me and many others too. You are not alone.), stick to fruits and veggies that will produce a lower insulin response. Berries, plums, watermelon, grapefruit, peaches/nectarines, cantaloupe, lemon/lime, oranges, honeydew, pears, guava, apricot, lettuce, bok choy, arugula, broccoli, carrots, tomatoes, garlic, radish, brussels sprouts, collard greens, kohlrabi, cauliflower, celery, avocado, mushrooms, asparagus, shallots, scallions, mustard greens, seaweed, cabbage, cucumbers, olives, swiss chard, leeks, onions, chives, turnip greens, okra, peppers, artichokes, spinach, and watercress. As you can see, there are still plenty of delicious options that have a low insulin response within our bodies. Those looking to gain weight or are insulin sensitive already have a little more freedom. Be wary of corn. As most of it is genetically modified and riddled with toxins. Look for organic, non-genetically modified corn.

I really cannot emphasize enough that it is highly unlikely that you will ever eat too many fruits or vegetables. Get a variety and try some of the weird ones. They are tasty and loaded with nutrients, antioxidants, polyphenols, and all sorts of things that are going to help improve our health. If you do not already know, these are the "superfoods" that help keep us healthy and young. Somewhere along the way, our society began to think that we knew better than mother nature. Thus, processed foods were born. But, I promise, mother nature knows what she is doing. Eat lots of vegetables and some fruit and reap the benefits of sustainable health.

When it comes to carbohydrates, the weird stuff is often the best for us. Look for organic produce to reduce exposure to toxins and increase the amount of nutrients you can pull from these foods. Conventional produce and many packaged goods containing wheat and other commodity crops often contains pesticides and other toxins that are detrimental to our health. We want to avoid these to keep our bodies running smoothly. Worse yet, conventional farming practices leak these toxins into the environment contaminating drinking water and the natural environments of many fish and other animals.

How much carbohydrates as well as the type is dictated largely by our goals. Those looking to lose weight, need a little bit less, and those looking to gain weight need a little bit more. If you are in the first category, your priority when building your plate should be vegetables. A little bit of low glycemic fruit can be added as well, but vegetables should be the focus. How much? Make a fist. That much. Try to get 3-4 fist-sized servings at every meal. Since you now know we do not actually need grains and starches, I will leave this to your best judgement. I encourage you to experiment. If you choose to incorporate these, stick to one cupped hand full. If you examine your cupped hand, you will notice that it is not very much. One cupped handful at dinner should be plenty. You may not want to eat them at all if you are not regularly exercising. If you are exercising, consume grains and starches following exercise since this is when we are most sensitive to insulin.

If you are an individual that is looking to gain weight, are a highly active person, or competitive athlete, you likely need a little more. We still want to time our consumption with the instances we are most insulin sensitive. Shoot for 2-3 cupped hands, but still at dinner or split between lunch and dinner. We want our breakfasts to be high in protein and fats so that we do not crash in the middle of the day. You may need more or less depending on your activity level. Experiment with how much along with the timing. If you are competing, do not experiment on the day of the competition. Off season training is the ideal time to experiment with different combinations. Make sure you are still eating as many vegetables and fruits as you can. As an athlete, you must maintain health to be able to compete at a high level. If you are looking for numbers, 4-7g/kg a day is a pretty good start. That can even be raised to 10g/kg a day if you are in a compressed schedule where multiple training sessions or games are happening in a single day.

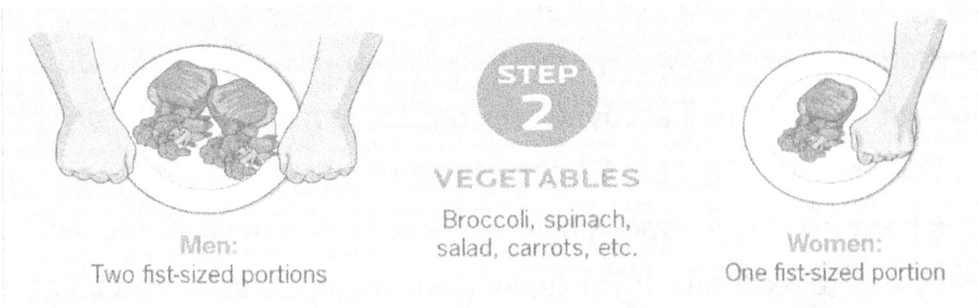

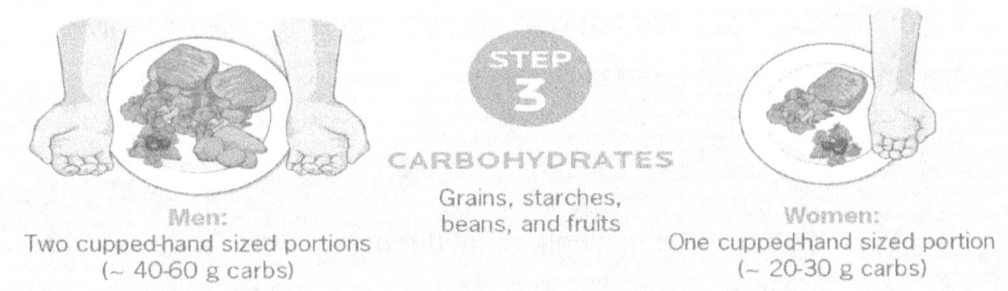

Carbohydrates

Now that we have an idea of why it is important to consume quality carbohydrates, we can get into how to implement the habit. The trick is to find what works best for you. We are all highly individual. I cannot tell you what is going to be best in your situation. That is something you must find on your own. A coach can help brainstorm ideas, but the execution falls on you. Use the notes section to brainstorm and track how different strategies work for you, and then work with your coach or accountability partner to really dial in what your best practice might be. Do not forget to continue the previous habits because they all work together. Focus on this habit for the next 4 weeks. Take more time if you need. Remember, we truly want this to become part of our lives.

Because of the variety in carbohydrate consumption based on our goals and other various factors, it is important that you work closely with your coach. If you are not working with a coach, take intricate notes and track your progress.

- Take it Slow - Pick a single meal during the week and add 2-3 servings (fist-sized) of quality sourced vegetables from the example above. Depending on your goals, also add 1-2 servings (cupped hands) of quality sourced grains or starches to one dinner. Use the notes section to notice how you feel.

- A Little More Challenging - Pick 3-4 meals during the week and add 2-3 servings (fist-sized) of quality sourced vegetables from the example above. Depending on your goals, also add 1-2 servings (cupped hands) of quality sourced grains or starches to 3-4 dinners. Use the notes section to notice how you feel.

- Ready for a Challenge - Add 2-3 servings (fist-sized) of quality sourced vegetables from the example above. Depending on your goals, also add 1-2 servings (cupped hands) of quality sourced grains or starches to 3-4 dinners. Use the notes section to notice how you feel.

Notes

General notes about the habit:

How are you planning on implementing this habit?

How ready, willing, and able are you to implement your strategy? (for a reminder on how to use this activity, see page 28)

What are some potential roadblocks you may face?

What are some strategies you can use prepare for these roadblocks?

What have you noticed about how you feel, think, or act after implementing this habit?

Which Pillars do you feel that this habit impacts? Why?

Any questions, comments, or concerns to bring up with your coach?

References

Asprey, D. (2020). *Superhuman: a bulletproof plan to age backward and maybe even live forever.* Harper Wave

Berardi, J., & Andrews, R. (2010). *The essentials of sport and exercise nutrition.* Precision Nutrition.

Bubbs, M. (2019). *Peak: The new science of athletic performance that is revolutionizing sports* Chelsea Green Publishing.

Connolly, F., & White, P. (2017). *Game changer* Simon and Schuster.

Harari, Y. N. (2014). *Sapiens: A brief history of humankind* Random House.

https://www.precisionnutrition.com/calorie-control-guide-infographic

Hyman, M. (2018). *Food: What the heck should I eat?* Hachette UK.

Hyman, M. (2020). *Food Fix: How to Save Our Health, Our Economy, Our Communities, and Our Planet -- One Bite at a Time.* Little, Brown Spark

LaValle, J. B., & Yale, S. L. (2004). *Cracking the metabolic code: The nine keys to peak health* Basic Health Publications, Inc.

Learney, P. (2014). *N1 nutritional programming: The fundamentals of nutritional programming.* ACA

Neth, B. J., & Craft, S. (2017). Insulin resistance and alzheimer's disease: Bioenergetic linkages. *Frontiers in Aging Neuroscience, 9,* 345.

Perlmutter, D. (2018). *Grain brain: The surprising truth about wheat, carbs, and sugar--your brain's silent killers* Hachette UK.

Saslow, L. R., Summers, C., Aikens, J. E., & Unwin, D. J. (2018). Outcomes of a digitally delivered low-carbohydrate type 2 diabetes self-management program: 1-year results of a single-arm longitudinal study. *JMIR Diabetes, 3*(3), e12.

Taubes, G. (2007). *Good calories, bad calories* Anchor.

Habit 8: Fats

Oh fats. The unfortunate macronutrient that shares its name with adipose tissue. Thanks to this fact along with some poor research studies and excellent politicking in the 1950's, fat is a scary and confusing subject for many people. So, hopefully, we can make it less scary and less confusing here. This is going to be a long one. So, buckle in. I will try to be brief, but it is critical we understand how important fats are to our well-being. Because the right fats are actually very beneficial for our health.

Fats are made up of carbon and hydrogen molecules joined together to make hydrocarbons. How these hydrocarbons are arranged dictate the type of fat. If hydrogen ions take up all the bonding sites within the chain of molecules, this is a saturated fat. These are semi-solid at room temperature such as butter, coconut oil, or cocoa butter. If only some of the hydrogen molecules are bonded, we have an unsaturated fat, and these are usually liquid at room temperature. This group can be broken down to monounsaturated fats (one free carbon), and polyunsaturated fats (multiple free carbons). When 3 fatty acids are combined, we get a triglyceride. This is the major storage form of fat within our bodies. Fat does not dissolve in water, so it needs a little help to be transported around our bodies to the places it is needed. So, to aid in this we have lipoproteins.

Very-low-density-lipoproteins (VLDL) carry new triglycerides from the liver to adipose tissue, low-density-lipoproteins (LDL) carry cholesterol to all cells within the body, and high-density-lipoproteins (HDL) bring fat and cholesterol from the cells back into the liver. We want our LDL to be large and buoyant. This is an excellent indicator of good health. HDL is often known as the good cholesterol. This is because it is responsible for clearing excess cholesterol from cells, like our arteries. In general, a high HDL is also a good indicator of good health. We want our LDL to be lower in order to decrease the potential for clogged arteries, but we also want to ensure that they are large and buoyant so they are capable of properly carrying our cholesterol without allowing a drop-offs to clog our arteries. If you have current bloodwork or are planning to get some soon, the ratio of HDL to LDL to shoot for is 3.5:1 for males. 5:1 is probably as high as you would like to see this go. For females, 3.4:1 is optimal with 4.4:1 being about as high as you would like to see that ratio.

Cholesterol is something that also gets a bad rap, but our bodies need cholesterol. Our sex hormones - testosterone, and estrogen - are created from cholesterol. Our glucocorticoids are also made from cholesterol. Our livers create most of the cholesterol within our bodies, and it tightly regulates the amount within the system. It has even been shown that the cholesterol we eat, such as from egg yolks, does not have a huge impact on the serum cholesterol (cholesterol within our blood). Not to mention fat is responsible for insulating our nerve cells and is the primary component of cell membranes. Our brains are also made up of 70% fat. Thus, the overall health of our brains, nerves, and cells could be drastically impacted by reducing fat intake by too much.

I previously mentioned that we need to have a balanced ratio of omega-3 fats to omega-6 fats. Omega-3 fats are essential because they reduce inflammation, contribute to cardiovascular function, nervous system function, immune health, and they help our cell membranes to be more fluid. This fluidity allows neurotransmitters to enter the cell and work their magic more easily. It also increases our insulin sensitivity. There are 3 main types of omega-3 fats: EPA, DHA, and ALA. EPA and DHA are mainly found from marine sources. ALA is mainly from plant sources and can be converted to EPA and DHA within our body. However, the conversion ratio is very poor. Thus, plant-based eaters should probably look for a good supplement containing EPA and DHA.

Omega- 6 fats are responsible for constricting our blood vessels, increasing inflammation, and causing blood clotting. These fats are found in similar fats as omega 3 fats and are very prevalent within industrially processed foods. We need omega-6 fats because blood clotting, and inflammation are great for healing. While we want to keep systemic inflammation down over the long term, an acute incidence requires these processes to be functioning properly for us to recover properly. A 3:1 or 2:1 ratio of omega-6 to omega-3 is what we should be shooting for. Currently, the typical western diet has a ratio somewhere between 10:1 and 20:1 which leads to unhealthy, long-term inflammation levels within our bodies.

We also need to talk about trans fats. Many of these fats are unnatural and are the result of the low-fat craze that took the United States by storm. Before we get into how that happened, let us quickly get into why we do not want trans fats or any industrial oil that does not occur naturally within our systems. Trans fats are created by pumping unsaturated fats and flowing hydrogen ions through it until it is solid at room temperature. This process is where the term hydrogenated oils come from. When consumed these fats do not fold easily, but instead are tightly packed into our cell membranes. Remember, we want these membranes to be fluid so things can go in and out. These fats are also known to decrease HDL, increase our own cholesterol production, compete with the essential fats for transport into cells, and worsen any fatty acid deficiencies we may have. Luckily, these fats are being phased out of all food products. Naturally occurring trans fats such as CLA do not have the same effect on our bodies, so we do not have to worry about them.

We can finally get into how the fat scare came about. Now, when I said poor research studies at the beginning of this habit, the studies themselves were not poor. The conclusions drawn from them did indeed show a correlation between saturated fat and cardiovascular disease. If you remember anything from high school, you may recall that correlation does not equal causation. There were many scientists at this time who suggested that more research was required to truly decipher whether saturated fats did indeed cause cardiovascular disease. But there was a very vocal individual leading the charge against saturated fats. The main thought being that saturated fats increase cholesterol, cholesterol increased risk of cardiovascular disease, and therefore, saturated fats increased the risk for cardiovascular disease. It is true that saturated fats do raise cholesterol. However, is this a bad thing? Does a higher level of cholesterol mean we are at risk for cardiovascular disease? Let us dig into some of the data out there.

Ancel Keys was quite vocal about the correlation between saturated fats and cardiovascular disease. He and many of his followers were the most published authors on the subject at the time, and their work mostly involved citing the work of their peers. They believed their hypothesis to be correct, and designed studies which help to bolster their theories. As Gary Taubes notes, this is exactly what the scientific method hopes to avoid. Unfortunately, it still happens. Contrary data took longer to collect and was mostly ignored once published.

You may recall that our ancestors were hunter-gatherers. Food was not always around, and much of what they ate consisted of animal meats, the remaining parts of the animal as nothing was wasted, and some fruits and vegetables on a good day. Long before we even knew what saturated fats were, we were consuming them, and we were living relatively healthy lives. In fact, aside from a rare case of a deadly disease or an attack by a predator, our ancestors lived a long time, and often died peacefully in their sleep. A deeper dive into the data shows that tribes and groups that followed a more hunter-gatherer type diet remained healthy despite high levels of fat content. It was not until these groups became more "westernized" that prevalence of disease began to rise. What is a "westernized" diet? It is very similar to what we see in our culture today: lots of grains, breads, and sugars. In multiple areas across the globe such as the Masai, Samburu, and Rendille tribes diabetes and cardiovascular disease were not a concern until western culture got its grip on the culture of these tribes.

A perfect example of contrary evidence to Keys' theories being ignored is the Framingham Study. Launched in 1950, this study was designed to observe a single community in order to draw out potential indicators that may increase the likelihood of cardiovascular disease for its members. 5,100 individuals participated in this study, and they underwent physicals and blood work. They were examined every 2 years to see who contracted cardiovascular disease. High blood pressure, abnormal electrocardiograms, obesity, smoking, and genes were all identified as indicators of increased risk of cardiovascular disease. In 1961 it was also found that high cholesterol was another indicator. Indeed, men who had cholesterol over 260 mg/dl were 5 times more likely to contract cardiovascular disease than those whose cholesterol had been under 200. This is often touted as indisputable proof that cholesterol is the culprit.

But that is not all there is to the story. As these men aged, those who had contracted cardiovascular disease were even more likely to have lower cholesterol, and there was little data to support the theory for women under 50, and there was no evidence at all for women over 50. This evidence failed to support the hypothesis of Keys. However, this information never got out. Gary Taubes, author of *Good Calories Bad Calories* notes, "George Mann, who left the Framingham Study in the early 1960s, recalled that the NIH administrators who funded the work refused to allow publication. Only in the late 1960s did the NIH biostatistician Tavia Gordon come across the data and decide they were worth writing up." He goes on to explain that fat consumption between individuals with cholesterol over 300, and those with cholesterol under 170 varied little in amount of type. In 1971, the investigators finally observed that cholesterol is not an indicator of cardiovascular disease. These findings are the same in virtually every single study of varying populations throughout the country and the world.

While Keys did jump the gun, it is important to note that he was simply trying to create a positive change on the lifestyle of Americans. Unfortunately, the fat scare and subsequent weaning from fat may have caused the current obesity and chronic disease epidemic we now face. It is also important to note that we need to let the scientific method run its course. We cannot draw conclusions from incomplete data, and we must be willing to change our minds when data does not support our theories. No drug or medicine could ever be approved by the methods which resulted in the low-fat craze, and dietary suggestions and recommendations should be treated the same. As Hippocrates once wisely stated, "Let food be thy medicine, and medicine thy food."

By now, hopefully you are no longer scared of fat, and understand that is an essential part of a healthy diet. We need the right fats for our bodies to function the way they are intended. In fact, higher fat diets (when the right fats are ingested) have been shown to reduce the risk of heart disease, diabetes, and obesity. Fats also help with absorption of some nutrients, so make sure to eat plenty of vegetables as well! Where do the right fats come from, and how much should we eat?

As with meats, and everything we eat, it is important we are getting quality sourced fats. If we are going to eat butter or milk, it should come from grass-fed cows. We learned about industrial cattle in the protein habit. The milk and dairy from healthy, grass-fed cows are also much more nutritious. Whole milk can be a great source of fat and protein. However, we do not really need it. We are the only mammals to drink milk past the infant stage, and about 70% of people cannot digest dairy. Whole milk is best for us since the other kinds are mostly the sugars left over and have been stripped of much of the nutrients. These types then need to be re-fortified of the important vitamins and nutrients the standard recommendations suggest we get from them. In fact, low fat milk has been linked to many health problems and higher rates of obesity. The same is true of things like yogurt. It can be healthy form grass-fed cows, but most products on the market come with added sugars that negate any positive effects.

To ensure we are getting a good ratio of omega-3 to omega-6, we need to ensure we are consuming grass-fed, grass-finished meats and wild caught seafood. Wild game is also a great source too, for all of you hunters out there. Omega-3 fats are also found in eggs, flaxseeds, algae, and walnuts. Omega-6 fats are found primarily in nuts, seeds, grains, beans, highly refined vegetable oils, and ultra-processed foods. That is not to say that we should avoid nuts, seeds, some grains, and some beans. Remember, we still need some omega-6 fats in our diets. However, we should avoid the highly refined vegetable oils (soybean oil, canola oil, corn oil, safflower oil, sunflower oil, palm oil, peanut oil, vegetable oil, vegetable shortening, margarine, and anything that isn't natural or is hydrogenated) and ultra-processed foods.

Highly refined vegetable and seed oils were never intended for consumption they were created to help lubricate machinery. I think it bears repeating that they were never intended for human consumption. It is best to stick with extra-virgin olive oil, coconut oil, ghee, grass-fed butter, and avocado oil. Remember we want to try and go organic when we can to ensure we are not risking exposure to pesticides and other toxic chemicals. When we cook with these oils, we need to stay below the smoke point as this is the point in which the fat begins to break down which then increases the amount oxidation and inflammation in our bodies when consumed. Avocado oil is great for high heats (520°F), coconut oil is great for low/medium heats (350°F), ghee is good for high heat (450°F), and olive oil is great for low/medium heats (325°F). When we use higher heats than the oils can handle, we increase oxidation (the same thing that happens when metal rusts) of the fats and inflammation within our bodies. If you're looking for a healthy salad topping, and a great way to get some healthy fats in the diet go for olive oil, walnut oil, almond oil, macadamia oil, sesame seed oil, tahini, flax oil, and hemp oil. These should not be cooked with. If you are looking for a snack, nut butters can be a good source of healthy fats too. Just be aware of things like added sugar. If you go with a nut butter, the only ingredient should be the nut itself. Raw and organic is typically the gold standard for nut butters. You will learn for other things to look out for like hidden sugars in the Pantry Shakedown Habit as well.

I even keep a picture of the chart below with me when I shop. I also sent it to my wife, so she has it handy as well. This can help you keep track of the fats we should be getting more of along with those we should work to avoid. I originally found it in *Deep Nutrition*, but the information is consistent across books and research alike. I hope that it is as helpful for you as it is for our family.

Good Fats	Bad Fats
Olive Oil	Canola Oil
Peanut Oil	Soy Oil
Butter	Sunflower Oil
Macadamia Nut Oil	Cottonseed Oil
Coconut Oil	Grapeseed Oil
Tallow	Safflower Oil
Palm Oil	Non-butter spreads

Now how much should we be eating? Luckily, we have our handy tool, our hands (corny pun definitely intended). Our thumbs are about the size of a portion of fat. We can shoot for 1-2 thumbs 3-4 times per day. For the number people out there, shoot for about 30% of Calories to come from fats. Do not go under 20%, and it is okay to go over 30%. For you Keto supporters this is great news. The ketogenic diet can be an excellent tool to increase insulin sensitivity and decrease body fat percentage. However, to maintain ketosis over a long period of time is difficult and can lead to some significant rebounding effects. Our bodies perform their best when they can use fat and carbohydrates for energy. So, if you are a keto believer, cycle in and out of ketosis for optimal health. Dave Asprey, founder of bulletproof and the individual that has brought the keto diet to light in recent days, has been on record saying just that. So, if you do not believe me, maybe his word will do it for you. This also prevents the rebounding effect and makes the results you see more long term. Plus, vegetables are carbohydrates, and we need to eat vegetables. So, cutting carbohydrates too low could potentially have some other negative side effects such as nutrient deficiencies.

Are you still with me? I did warn you that this might be a long one. By now you should have a better understanding of why we should be giving fats more love in our diets.

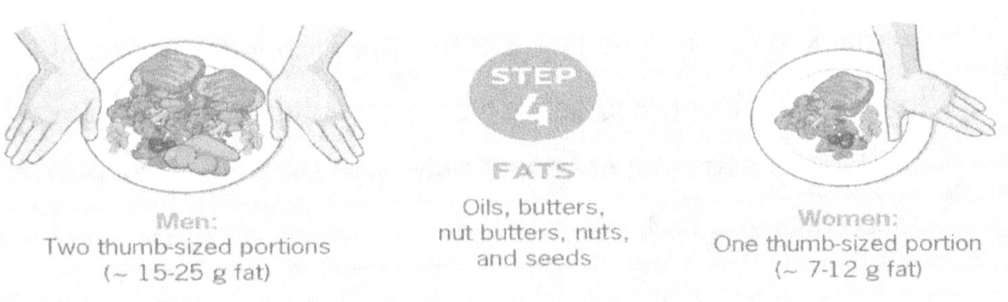

Fats

Now that we have an idea of why it is important to consume quality fats, we can get into how to implement the habit. The trick is to find what works best for you. We are all highly individual. I cannot tell you what is going to be best in your situation. That is something you must find on your own. A coach can help brainstorm ideas, but the execution falls on you. Use the notes section to brainstorm and track how different strategies work for you, and then work with your coach or accountability partner to really dial in what your best practice might be. Do not forget to continue the previous habits because they all work together. Focus on this habit for the next 4 weeks. Take more time if you need. Remember, we truly want this to become part of our lives.

- Take it Slow - Pick a single meal during the week and add 1-2 servings (thumbs) of quality sourced fats from the example above. Maybe add a side salad to dinner topped with one of the oils. Or maybe add some grass-fed butter to your grass-fed steak. Or maybe just eat some nuts. Use the notes section to notice how you feel.

- A Little More Challenging - Pick 3-4 meals during the week and add 1-2 servings (thumbs) of quality sourced fats from the example above. Use the notes section to notice how you feel.

- Ready for a Challenge - Add 1-2 servings (thumbs) of quality sourced fats from the example above to every meal. Use the notes section to notice the difference in how you feel.

Notes

General notes about the habit:

How are you planning on implementing this habit?

How ready, willing, and able are you to implement your strategy? (for a reminder on how to use this activity, see page 28)

What are some potential roadblocks you may face?

What are some strategies you can use prepare for these roadblocks?

What have you noticed about how you feel, think, or act after implementing this habit?

Which Pillars do you feel that this habit impacts? Why?

Any questions, comments, or concerns to bring up with your coach?

References

Asprey, D. (2018). *Game changers: What leaders, innovators, and mavericks do to win at life* HarperCollins.

Berardi, J., & Andrews, R. (2010). *The essentials of sport and exercise nutrition.* Precision Nutrition.

Bubbs, M. (2019). *Peak: The new science of athletic performance that is revolutionizing sports* Chelsea Green Publishing.

Connolly, F., & White, P. (2017). *Game changer* Simon and Schuster.

Harari, Y. N. (2014). *Sapiens: A brief history of humankind* Random House.

Hoenselaar, R. (2012). Saturated fat and cardiovascular disease: The discrepancy between the scientific literature and dietary advice. *Nutrition, 28*(2), 118-123.

https://www.precisionnutrition.com/calorie-control-guide-infographic

Hyman, M. (2018). *Food: What the heck should I eat?* Hachette UK.

LaValle, J. B., & Yale, S. L. (2004). *Cracking the metabolic code: The nine keys to peak health* Basic Health Publications, Inc.

Learney, P. (2014). *N1 nutritional programming: The fundamentals of nutritional programming.* ACA

Malhotra, A., Redberg, R. F., & Meier, P. (2017). Saturated fat does not clog the arteries: Coronary heart disease is a chronic inflammatory condition, the risk of which can be effectively reduced from healthy lifestyle interventions. *BMJ Publishing Group Ltd and British Association of Sport and Exercise Medicine,*

Shanahan, C. (2017). *Deep nutrition: Why your genes need traditional food.* Flatiron Books.

Taubes, G. (2007). *Good calories, bad calories* Anchor.

Verstegen, M., & Williams, P. (2014). *Every day is game day: Train like the pros with a no-holds-barred exercise and nutrition plan for peak performance* Penguin.

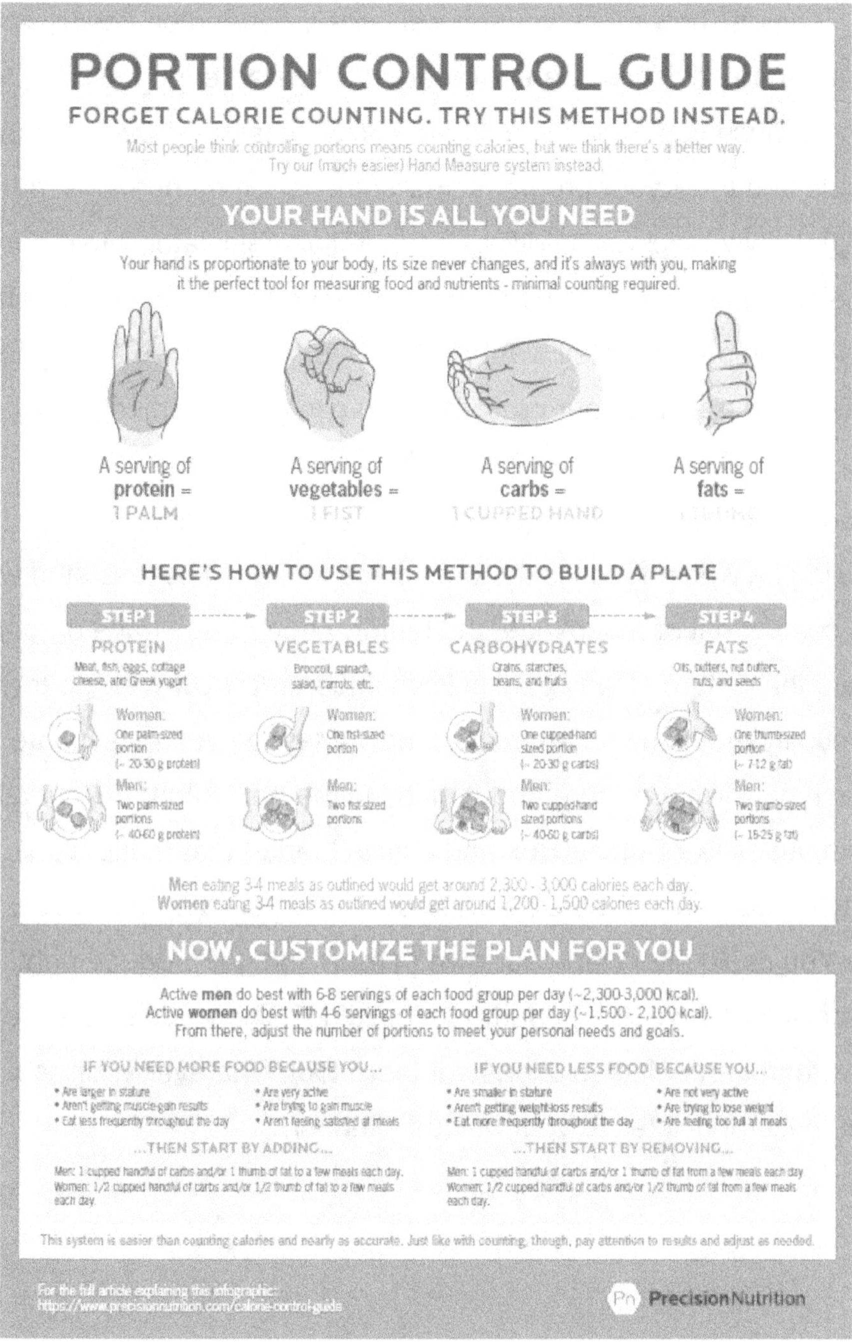

PORTION CONTROL GUIDE
FORGET CALORIE COUNTING. TRY THIS METHOD INSTEAD.
Most people think controlling portions means counting calories, but we think there's a better way. Try our (much easier) Hand Measure system instead.

YOUR HAND IS ALL YOU NEED

Your hand is proportionate to your body, its size never changes, and it's always with you, making it the perfect tool for measuring food and nutrients - minimal counting required.

A serving of protein = 1 PALM
A serving of vegetables = 1 FIST
A serving of carbs = 1 CUPPED HAND
A serving of fats = 1 THUMB

HERE'S HOW TO USE THIS METHOD TO BUILD A PLATE

STEP 1
PROTEIN
Meat, fish, eggs, cottage cheese, and Greek yogurt
Women: One palm-sized portion (~ 20-30 g protein)
Men: Two palm-sized portions (~ 40-60 g protein)

STEP 2
VEGETABLES
Broccoli, spinach, salad, carrots, etc.
Women: One fist-sized portion
Men: Two fist-sized portions

STEP 3
CARBOHYDRATES
Grains, starches, beans, and fruits
Women: One cupped-hand sized portion (~ 20-30 g carbs)
Men: Two cupped-hand sized portions (~ 40-60 g carbs)

STEP 4
FATS
Oils, butters, nut butters, nuts, and seeds
Women: One thumb-sized portion (~ 7-12 g fat)
Men: Two thumb-sized portions (~ 15-25 g fat)

Men eating 3-4 meals as outlined would get around 2,300 - 3,000 calories each day.
Women eating 3-4 meals as outlined would get around 1,200 - 1,500 calories each day.

NOW, CUSTOMIZE THE PLAN FOR YOU

Active men do best with 6-8 servings of each food group per day (~2,300-3,000 kcal).
Active women do best with 4-6 servings of each food group per day (~1,500 - 2,100 kcal).
From there, adjust the number of portions to meet your personal needs and goals.

IF YOU NEED MORE FOOD BECAUSE YOU...
• Are larger in stature
• Aren't getting muscle-gain results
• Eat less frequently throughout the day
• Are very active
• Are trying to gain muscle
• Aren't feeling satisfied at meals

...THEN START BY ADDING...
Men: 1 cupped handful of carbs and/or 1 thumb of fat to a few meals each day.
Women: 1/2 cupped handful of carbs and/or 1/2 thumb of fat to a few meals each day.

IF YOU NEED LESS FOOD BECAUSE YOU...
• Are smaller in stature
• Aren't getting weight-loss results
• Eat more frequently throughout the day
• Are not very active
• Are trying to lose weight
• Are feeling too full at meals

...THEN START BY REMOVING...
Men: 1 cupped handful of carbs and/or 1 thumb of fat from a few meals each day
Women: 1/2 cupped handful of carbs and/or 1/2 thumb of fat from a few meals each day.

This system is easier than counting calories and nearly as accurate. Just like with counting, though, pay attention to results and adjust as needed.

For the full article explaining this infographic:
https://www.precisionnutrition.com/calorie-control-guide

Pn Precision Nutrition

Overall, how much you eat will largely depend on your goals. These general guidelines are a great point to start experimenting to find how much you need in your situation. Play around with your own portions and track your progress. For some recommendations, head to https://www.precisionnutrition.com/nutrition-calculator (I told you Precision Nutrition had some awesome tools) to get a solid baseline from the portions you may want to start with. From there, track your progress. By tracking your progress, you can quickly adjust your portion size. Fortunately, we always have our hands with us, so portioning out food according to our goals can be relatively easy. Focusing on whole foods is the best place to start. The less stuff we have coming out of a package, the better. I hope that I have properly painted the picture of why quality is so important. However, go for the best quality that you can afford right now. Maybe even investigate CSA's (you will learn more about these in the next habit) in your area or companies like ButcherBox and Misfits Market that make high quality products accessible and affordable delivered right to your door! You could also start your own garden and get produce right in your backyard. Live in an apartment building? There are some pretty good urban gardening solutions out there too! Whatever your goals, adapt these principles to your unique situation.

Section IV: Putting It All Together

Your mindset is in the right place, your sleep is on point, and your support system has been built. You have an excellent understanding of where food should come from and what you should be eating. You are likely already feeling better and seeing results. You are still crushing it! Keep it up! Give yourself a pat on the back

Now we need to put it all together. We must have an environment suitable for our new lifestyle, and we must learn how to create meals. Although we should be focusing on whole foods, we will also go over what to look for on a nutrition label, and how to pick healthy snacks.

Habit 9: Pantry Shakedown

Before we get started on making our meals, our pantries likely need some work. What should our pantry consist of? How do we read nutrition labels to make sure we are eating the right things? These are some of the things we are going to talk about within this habit.

We will start with labels. In a perfect world, companies would not even be able to use the ingredients that are making us sick. However, we do not live in that world right now. So, we have to be able to read nutrition labels. The labels themselves are not super important. They give a breakdown of nutrient and Calorie content. Have you noticed that I have not once mentioned Calorie counting? I am of the belief that it is unnecessary (there are some circumstances where it would be beneficial). When we focus on whole foods, tune in to our bodies and hunger cues, and use the hand portion guide, we are usually right where we need to be.

What we are really concerned about from the nutrition label are the ingredients. Do not be fooled by branding and marketing techniques that label foods as "health" foods and other labels such as organic, gluten-free, vegan, keto, or anything else that might be used to catch your attention. In packaged products, these labels are not important. The ingredients list cannot lie. Ingredients are always listed from greatest to least amount contained within the food.

What are you looking for in an ingredients list? Foods we recognize, short ingredients list, and nothing that sounds like it should not be consumed by any animal. Refined white flour (pastas, breads, bagels, cereals, pretzels, muffins, etc.) should be consumed minimally if at all. Products with added sugar, vegetable oil, soybean oil, or any hydrogenated oils get the boot as well (refer to the fat habit for the complete list). Companies are especially sneaky with sugar. Sugar comes in the form of sugar, high-fructose corn syrup, corn syrup, malt, maltodextrin, any kind of syrup, honey, and almost anything that ends in -ose. Products with these in the first 5 ingredients have a lot per serving, but if it is listed at all, we want to work to avoid it as best we can. Sugar does a lot of damage to our bodies. Do not opt for artificial sweeteners as they can disrupt our gut microbiome, and they can cause inflammation. Sugar alcohols such as xylitol and erythritol can be healthy. They minimally impact blood sugar and insulin, and they benefit our gut microbiome too. However, some people have issues with gas and bloating. Drinks other than water, coffee, or tea should be mostly avoided, and make sure there is nothing added to them.

Another sneaky place toxins slip into our body is "natural flavors". These "flavors", organic or not, are a loose term that gives companies near free reign on what they put in their products. Do all companies use this to put toxic things in their foods? Probably not.

However, as a general rule of them, avoid natural flavorings in order to avoid risking exposure to toxins.

Fried foods like chips, and anything with MSG or soy as the main source of protein should also get replaced. Frozen meals that need to be microwaved and contain ingredients we do not recognize need to go.

To put it simply: if it is not something we talked about in the previous habits, we probably do not need to be consuming it. You might have already started pruning your pantry naturally as you learned more about the foods we should be eating in Section III. If not, now is the time.

What can we keep around? Spices are excellent but remember that quality matters. Organic vegetables and fruits. Local, unfiltered honey is also a decent way to get your sweet fix. Just do not go overboard with it. Remember we want to stick to the low glycemic list for the most part. Grass-fed beef and lamb, pasture-raised pork, poultry, and eggs, wild-caught small fish like salmon, grass-fed butter or ghee, grass-fed whole milk without any additives, and grass-fed yogurt and kefir without added sugar are all things we want to keep around. Whole grains such as quinoa, millet, teff, amaranth, black rice, and brown rice. Remember, we like the weird stuff. One weird type of food we have gotten away from in our society is fermented foods. These feed the good bacteria in our gut. By now you should understand that this is a great thing for our health. We can also add some of the smaller beans like lentils, adzuki, and navy beans.

Condiments are also an essential part of a healthy kitchen. We could always make our own, but that is not always an option. The same rules apply for condiments. Organic is best, and only if there are no additives. We also should be able to recognize all the ingredients on the label. Olive oil is great for salads. Prymal Kitchen also has a tremendous selection of healthy salad dressings. I do not want you to think everything is off limits. In fact, there are healthy versions of almost all products out there. We just need to know what we are looking for! Now that you have an understanding of what to look for in the ingredients list, you will be able to pick these out.

It is important to always remember that organic products are less likely to be contaminated with pesticides and be more nutritious. Furthermore, it is estimated that we process 60 tons of food throughout our lives. This can be a great opportunity to ensure we are getting the proper nutrients, or it could be an added strain to our detoxifying systems. These toxins can impact our hormone systems which can then affect our ability to recover, perform, or can increase our body fat percentage. We must be cognizant of the potential impact our food can have on our bodies. The impact can be both positive or negative.

We are even learning that organic may not be enough. Current agricultural practices have led to the destruction of our land and a lack of nutrient density in our foods. In fact, the UN estimates that we have 60 years of harvests remaining if we do not make a shift. Cue regenerative agriculture. Regenerative agriculture is the process of restoring soil and sequestering carbon from the atmosphere in order to put it back into the soil to encourage a diverse population of biological organisms in the soil. Food, including meats, grown using regenerative agricultural practices are healthier for us, help to reverse the effects of climate change, and require less inputs from farmers. It utilizes practices that work in conjunction with natural processes instead of trying to force nature to bend to our will. Overall, this is where we want our agricultural system to head. For a look at the benefits and why we need to make this switch, check out *Kiss the Ground* on Netflix. Or, head to https://www.kissthegroundmovie.com to learn more.

What if we cannot afford organic produce? Companies such as Aldi are making organic foods more affordable. Even the bigger grocery chains like Kroger, Publix, and Walmart are expanding the sections which contain healthy food options. Of course, there is always Whole Foods, but there are some other things we can do too. The first is to vote with our dollars. When we are willing to pay for quality products, it forces companies to re-evaluate the products they put out in the market. But you just told me you cannot afford them.

Buy seasonal. Seasonal groceries are abundant, and therefore carry a lower price. If you are not sure what is seasonal, ask someone in the store. If for some reason they will not help, a quick internet search should be able to solve the mystery.

Go local. If you have a farmer's market nearby, go get your produce and groceries there. Smaller farms often use organic practices, but they cannot afford the organic label. Their products are top notch, and very affordable. Plus, you can simply ask what methods they use to farm, and if they are adding pesticides or other toxins, move on to the next vendor. Farmer's markets are a great place to get your groceries if it is something available to you. Many of these small farm's also utilize a community sourced agriculture (CSA) program. This allows you to pay a monthly fee, and you get an assortment of the farm's products at no additional costs. When the farm does well, you get more, and if they are struggling, you get a little less. This gives you skin in the game, and a vested interest in how your local farms are doing.

These same strategies can be used to buy grass-fed, grass-finished meats. You can even use a delivery service like ButcherBox to get high quality meat delivered right to your door. This all sounds expensive. However, we overconsume meat as a society. By cutting back and thinking of meat more as a condiment (a condi-meat as Dr. Hyman likes to say), we save money on meat. Then we can focus on purchasing other high-quality items like produce and other pantry staples.

What if farmer's markets are not an option? Luckily, there is a list called the "dirty dozen" and "clean fifteen". This is a list of foods most likely to be contaminated by toxins (dirty dozen), and most likely to not contain toxins (clean 15). These lists are provided by the Environmental Working Group (https://www.ewg.org/foodnews/). The lists change every year, but as of writing this the lists look like this:

Dirty Dozen	**Clean 15**
Strawberries	Avocados
Spinach	Sweet Corn (Often GMO)
Kale	Pineapples
Nectarines	Sweet Peas (frozen)
Apples	Onions
Grapes	Papayas (often GMO – be careful)
Peaches	Eggplants
Cherries	Asparagus
Pears	Kiwis
Tomatoes	Cabbages
Celery	Cauliflower

Potatoes

Hot Peppers

Cantaloupes

Broccoli

Mushrooms

Honeydew Melons

As you can see, there are still plenty of options if you cannot go full organic at this time. The more color and variety we can get, the better. We want most of our food to come from whole food sources. So, our fridges should be filled with colorful options.

What about snacks? Do we even need them? Probably not. But it is important to prevent a food emergency if we want to ensure success. So, raw and unsalted nuts are loaded with nutrients and a great way to add some healthy fats. Nut butters without additives are another great snack. As cliche as it sounds, vegetables and fruits are the absolute best snack. Loaded with nutrients, and easy to take on the go. Keep some hummus around, and you have an excellent alternative to chips and dip. Really, any dip goes well with vegetables. Guacamole, salsa, spinach and artichoke, and anything else you can think of likely taste great with some vegetables. You can make your own, or you can buy some. Just make sure you are checking the ingredient list! Baked vegetable chips are also pretty good. Any of these can be options for a snack. Remember, we want to stick with whole foods whenever it is possible. If you absolutely cannot take any of these on the go. Bulletproof bars and Perfect Food bars are both healthier alternatives than your typical protein or granola bars. Epic also has some good tasting snack foods, and a plethora of other things such as fats for cooking with. Remember to check the ingredient labels on other things that you may want to try. This is by no means an all-encompassing list.

We are also going to need to make sure the things we use to cook are not adding any toxins to our foods. For storage, eating, and packing. We should try to stick with glass. Plastics contain BPA, and even if they are BPA free, they often contain some of BPA's close relatives. So, it is best we work to phase these out of our pantries. For pots and pans, stainless steel or ceramic is going to be our best chance to avoid toxins slipping into our foods. You do not have to go out and get them right now if you do not have them. Maybe work to create a plan to slowly start acquiring them. A skillet is another good option, but make sure it does not have a nonstick coating. In fact, we want to avoid the nonstick coating in our sheet pans and anything else we cook with as well. A pressure cooker can also be a great tool to quickly whip up some meals. Plastic containers and utensils, nonstick coatings, and other toxins inhibit our ability absorb nutrients. So, even if we are getting the highest quality groceries, we may be negating those benefits from our choice of containers, utensils, and cookware. Chances are that your kitchen is already set for healthy cooking aside from a few minor details, so do not stress about this part too much. The big-ticket items are things with nonstick coating.

A quick thought on microwaves. Microwaves denature proteins and can increase oxidation in our bodies. Sometimes it just makes food taste funny too. I am not saying do not ever microwave anything, but maybe reduce the amount you are using one. Plus, we talked about how starches become even better for us when they are cooked and cooled. Try leftovers cold. I get a lot of crazy looks, but honestly, I prefer it.

Pay attention as you start to implement some of these strategies. You may notice a psychological benefit, and you will likely start to feel better overall. The quality of our food matters. If we want to be healthy, our food needs to come from healthy sources.

All of this is not to say your kitchen needs to be perfect. If you like to have ice cream occasionally, keep it around. Maybe you have the self-control to only eat a candy bar or a bag of chips on special occasions. That is impressive, and I wish I had that kind of ability. If it becomes something you consume too regularly and prevents you from reaching your goals, it might be time to come up with another strategy. For most of us, we are more apt to eat something when we see it. So, it might be best to avoid keeping the things we know are not going to help us reach our goals in our kitchens. I cannot tell you what will work best in your situation. That is for you to decide as you experiment with different strategies. Look for some of the red flags you learned about the next time you are shopping. You may be surprised at what some of your favorite foods contain.

Pantry Shakedown

Now that you understand what to keep around, we can get into how to implement the habit. The trick is to find what works best for you. We are all highly individual. I cannot tell you what is going to be best in your situation. That is something you must find on your own. A coach can help brainstorm ideas, but the execution falls on you. Use the notes section to brainstorm and track how different strategies work for you, and then work with your coach or accountability partner to really dial in what your best practice might be. Do not forget to continue the previous habits because they all work together. Focus on this habit for the next 4 weeks. Take more time if you need. Remember, we truly want this to become part of our lives.

- Take it Slow - Pick a single item from your pantry or fridge and read the food label. If it does not meet the criteria we discussed above, kick it to the curb. Do this once per week. If you need to take things extra slow, replace items with healthier alternatives as you run out of them.

- A Little More Challenging - Pick 5-10 items from your pantry or fridge and read the food label. If it does not meet the criteria we discussed above, kick it to the curb. Start to experiment with organic produce. Do this once per week.

- Ready for a Challenge - Completely overhaul your kitchen. Get rid of all the items with unhealthy additives and replace them with healthy alternatives. Your fridge is colorful, and everything is quality sourced.

Notes

General notes about the habit:

How are you planning on implementing this habit?

How ready, willing, and able are you to implement your strategy? (for a reminder on how to use this activity, see page 28)

What are some potential roadblocks you may face?

What are some strategies you can use prepare for these roadblocks?

What have you noticed about how you feel, think, or act after implementing this habit?

Which Pillars do you feel that this habit impacts? Why?

Any questions, comments, or concerns to bring up with your coach?

References

Berardi, J., & Andrews, R. (2010). *The essentials of sport and exercise nutrition*. Precision Nutrition.

Bubbs, M. (2019). *Peak: The new science of athletic performance that is revolutionizing sports* Chelsea Green Publishing.

Connolly, F., & White, P. (2017). *Game changer* Simon and Schuster.

Gundry, S. R. (2018). *The plant paradox cookbook: 100 delicious recipes to help you lose weight, heal your gut, and live lectin-free* HarperCollins.

https://www.kissthegroundmovie.com

Hyman, M. (2018). *Food: What the heck should I eat?* Hachette UK.

Hyman, M. (2020). *Food Fix: How to Save Our Health, Our Economy, Our Communities, and Our Planet -- One Bite at a Time.* Little, Brown Spark

LaValle, J. B., & Yale, S. L. (2004). *Cracking the metabolic code: The nine keys to peak health* Basic Health Publications, Inc.

Perlmutter, D. (2018). *Grain brain: The surprising truth about wheat, carbs, and sugar--your brain's silent killers* Hachette UK.

Sani, J. (2018). *Making healthy taste good: kick sugar for good, spike your food with health & flavor.* Jason Sani.

Shanahan, C. (2016). *Deep Nutrition: Why Your Genes Need Traditional Food.* Flatiron Books

Taleb, N. N. (2020). *Skin in the game: Hidden asymmetries in daily life* Random House Trade Paperbacks.

Habit 10: Home Cooked Meals

I have good news. You are in the home stretch now. This habit is simple. Cook your meals at home. Home cooked meals will always be better for us than food from fast food or other restaurants. When we cook food at home, we can control exactly what we are putting into it. There are even healthy alternatives to some of our favorite desserts too. Not to mention cooking at home can be a great tool to strengthen relationships and just have fun. If we look at many of the healthiest areas in the world, they have a connection with their food. Home cooked meals are all about connection. Connection with each other and connection with our food. Enjoying a meal with loved ones after preparing a healthy meal filled with love is a truly gratifying experience. I love cooking for my wife. I even tell her it is my love language, and it is something I hope you come to love as well.

If you have some experience cooking, this step is easy. Use your newly stocked pantry, pick what you want to eat, use the portion guide to get your servings, and then spice it up with different spices. Not a master chef? That is okay. I am not either. However, I can follow some basic instructions, and you can too. I am not going to break down the intricacies of cooking. Quite frankly, I do not know them. I am however going to help you plan your meals, give advice on picky eaters, and provide some places you can get some great recipes from.

When we cook at home, we can control the ingredients in both quality and quantity. We also have the potential to turn our favorite food items into healthy alternatives. There are ways to do it with foods like pizza, cookies, and just about anything you could imagine. With cooking at home, there is nearly no limit to what we can turn into healthy foods that ultimately help us reach our goals. Healthy foods can also taste delicious when we prepare them properly.

We can start with what our meals should consist of. We talked about it a little bit, but we will get into a little more detail here. For breakfast we want high protein and fat content. This prevents an insulin spike first thing in the morning. These foods also help to keep us full longer and prevent a crash a few hours after eating. I am sure you can recall that afternoon crash after a breakfast consisting of highly refined carbohydrates. You are not alone. It happens to all of us. High fat, high protein breakfasts are a great way to get our days started on the right foot. An easy way to do this is meat (to include eggs) and nuts. You should also throw in some vegetables and you could include a little bit of low glycemic fruit like berries. This adds variety and plenty of nutrients. Remember, the more vegetables and fruit we can get in, the more of the good stuff like polyphenols, antioxidants, and other nutrients we get. If you need something on the go, try making food ahead of time. You can also try making a smoothie, but I do suggest switching the meat for a protein powder. I am not sure how good that smoothie would be. Protein powder, fruits, veggies, your favorite nut butter, some water, and you are good to go. Breakfast on the move. It is still important to slow down though. Remember, it takes time for our bodies to recognize we are full.

We are going to go to dinner next. Dinner should consist of more veggies, meat, and quality starches or grains. You may recall how much starches or grains you use can vary depending on your goals. If you are not very active, you likely do not need much if any at all. Or maybe you limit it to a couple times per week. That is up to you. If you are active or an athlete, time your starches and grains with your activity levels. This allows your body to shuttle the sugar (since these things ultimately get broken down into sugar) into the muscles rapidly. Experiment with the content, use your hands to guide portions, and notice how you feel.

Now to the reason we skipped to dinner: Leftovers. Leftovers are a tremendous way to have a great lunch the next day. Simply cook a little bit extra, and now you do not have to worry about what you are going to eat for lunch. You can also always make lunches ahead of time. A salad is a great lunch option because it is quick, simple, and it is easy to pack away. Any meal can be prepped ahead of time for a healthy lunch. I have just found that leftovers are a good way to avoid the potential time cost of meal prepping.

Not sure where to start when picking recipes, or do you want some new ideas and inspiration? Try a service like Blue Apron or Hello Fresh. They deliver pre planned meals right to your door. All you need to do is follow directions. Most of their recipes and ingredients are things that we would never even think of using. It is a great way to try new things and broaden your culinary horizons. Most of their ingredients are of high quality too. But anything that is not, you can just make a quick substitution thanks to your pantry shakedown. The bad news is you do not really get leftovers. However, you can use something like this for a period to gain plenty of recipe options, and then begin to make them on your own when you can plan for leftovers.

What about those picky eaters? Get them involved! Have them pick between different vegetable options. Let them help with preparation. This gives them a vested interest in what the family eats. They become an active part of what the family is eating which gives them skin in the game. They can then recognize the hard work that went into the preparation of the family meal. It builds stronger relationships and helps build their own bit of healthy habits too. Remember to be patient with them. Recognize that they are likely trying things they have never tried before, and that is not easy.

Now where do we get our recipes from? I already mentioned Blue Apron and Hello Fresh. We have a binder full of them we still turn to. You can also go to their website for some of their recipes too. Here are some of my favorite cookbooks:

- *The Plant Paradox Family Cookbook*
- *The Grain Brain Cookbook*
- *Making Healthy Taste Good*

You can also use recipes from your favorite cookbook. Simply switch out the less than ideal ingredients. Pinterest is another great place to find some recipe ideas. Be careful with processed ingredients and remember your previous habits.

One key way to save money and ensure your shopping experience goes smoothly is planning ahead. We do this in other areas such as exercise and in business. Why should our meals be any different? Prior to going shopping, plan a menu. This does not have to be a day by day meal by meal menu. Instead, it is just a selection of meals and snacks you would like that week. Get everyone who will be eating and cooking involved (this helps with the picky eaters too). Once the meals are ready to go, plan out the ingredients needed. You may even break those down by section of the grocery store. Whatever works best for you. Then, the only thing left to do is go shopping and check items off the list. This eliminates the mindless wandering and guessing what ingredients you need. It also reduces the potential for last second purchases. You also probably want to avoid doing the shopping hungry. That is a quick way to get off track. Remember, if you fail to plan, you are planning to fail. So, set yourself up for success and plan your trip prior to going shopping.

You might be curious about fasting or time restricted eating. Like anything, it is a tool that can be used depending on your situation. There have been numerous benefits found from these things, but they can be quite difficult. Society has told us that we need to eat 3-4 times every day. Is that true? Our ancestors certainly did not do that. If these are things you feel you may benefit from, experiment with them. Notice how you feel. You may find that you consume more later in the day. Or you might find that it works really well for you when you practice time restricted eating. The choice is always yours. Should you experiment with it and not like it, you can always go back, but it is also totally cool to not even worry about these things. If you are an athlete, or in a very physical profession, I would suggest avoiding fasting and time restricted eating. You want your energy stores filled if you want to be able to perform at a high level.

Home Cooked Meals

Now that you better understand how to tackle home cooked meals, we can get into how to implement the habit. The trick is to find what works best for you. We are all highly individual. I cannot tell you what is going to be best in your situation. That is something you must find on your own. A coach can help brainstorm ideas, but the execution falls on you. Use the notes section to brainstorm and track how different strategies work for you, and then work with your coach or accountability partner to really dial in what your best practice might be. Do not forget to continue the previous habits because they all work together. Focus on this habit for the next 4 weeks. Take more time if you need. Remember, we truly want this to become part of our lives.

- Take it Slow - Pick a single meal during the week and make it from home. Try to incorporate those picky eaters if you have any. If you are having trouble picking a recipe, pick one of your favorites, and make it with healthy ingredients. Notice if your food makes you feel differently than your normal meal selection.

- A Little More Challenging - Pick 2-4 meals during the week and make it yourself. Try to incorporate those picky eaters if you have any. Notice if your food makes you feel differently than your normal meal selection.

- Ready for a Challenge - Make all your meals yourself. Try to incorporate those picky eaters if you have any. Notice if your food makes you feel differently than your normal meal selection.

Notes

General notes about the habit:

How are you planning on implementing this habit?

How ready, willing, and able are you to implement your strategy? (for a reminder on how to use this activity, see page 28)

What are some potential roadblocks you may face?

What are some strategies you can use prepare for these roadblocks?

What have you noticed about how you feel, think, or act after implementing this habit?

Which Pillars do you feel that this habit impacts? Why?

Any questions, comments, or concerns to bring up with your coach?

References

Bubbs, M. (2019). *Peak: The new science of athletic performance that is revolutionizing sports* Chelsea Green Publishing.

Gundry, S. R. (2018). *The plant paradox cookbook: 100 delicious recipes to help you lose weight, heal your gut, and live lectin-free* HarperCollins.

Perlmutter, D. (2014). *The grain brain cookbook* Little Brown & Company.

Perlmutter, D. (2018). *Grain brain: The surprising truth about wheat, carbs, and sugar--your brain's silent killers* Hachette UK.

Hyman, M. (2020). *Food Fix: How to Save Our Health, Our Economy, Our Communities, and Our Planet -- One Bite at a Time.* Little, Brown Spark

Sani, J. (2018). *Making healthy taste good: kick sugar for good, spike your food with health & flavor.* Jason Sani.

Taleb, N. N. (2020). *Skin in the game: Hidden asymmetries in daily life* Random House Trade Paperbacks.

Verstegen, M., & Williams, P. (2014). *Every day is game day: Train like the pros with a no-holds-barred exercise and nutrition plan for peak performance* Penguin.

Habit 11: Move

You may find it odd that as a Strength and Conditioning Coach I waited until near the end of this whole thing to bring up exercise. Well there is a reason for that. Exercise has some tremendous benefits which we will discuss here. But the reason it is near the end is because no matter how much we exercise, if the rest of our habits are not in place, we are not very likely to see the results we are looking for. The fact of the matter is this: we cannot exercise our way out of a bad diet. Balanced hormones, internal systems, and food quality all play a huge role in optimizing our health, but exercise can only take us so far in reaching our goals. Does it help? Sure, but only when we work to get everything else in our bodies working optimally too. Not to mention that the chances are you were also already exercising are high. You are reading a book about optimizing health. I do not think it would be a huge gamble on my part to assume that some form of exercise is going on in your life (if I am wrong, I will consider myself wise in avoiding gambling altogether).

You may believe that if you want to lose weight, you have to do tons of cardio, and if you want to gain weight, you should be lifting lots of weights. Well I am here to tell you that is not the case. Running is a very high impact activity, and the repetitive movements and impacts that occur during running can cause a lot of damage to our joints as well as our bodies increasing the possibility of injury. Mike Boyle notes the typical cycle of adults who pick up running to lose weight looks something like this: run → injury → rehab, and then the cycle repeats itself. He also notes that it is like slamming your hand in a car door. This is not something you are likely to repeat, so why do we continue to go back to exercise methods that continue to hurt us? I have been caught in this cycle myself, and not just running. Many popular exercises have made their way out of my programs for this exact reason. It is about time we stop the cycle. If you are worried about getting too bulky or putting on too much weight from strength training, it takes a very specific type of training and nutrition protocol to elicit this type of growth. Simply starting a strength training program is not going to make you look like the Hulk. This is true for males and females.

Furthermore, strength training is actually very good for losing weight. When we participate in high intensity exercise our bodies go through a litany of healthy adaptations. We become more insulin sensitive, our growth hormones increase, we sleep better at night, our bones and connective tissues get stronger (which is why it's important we strength train if we are runners), our body composition improves, our brains are more efficient thanks to increased levels of brain derived neurotrophic factor, our muscles get more efficient, our workouts are more efficient, and we actually burn more Calories thanks to something called EPOC. We will talk about EPOC in a second but let us discuss some other benefits of strength training.

What is a great indicator of independence in old age? Muscle strength. Why? Let us think critically about it. In old age, we are typically weaker, a little more fragile, and less mobile. These are all factors that strength training improves. This means that by incorporating strength training (along with the other habits we learned about) as we continue to age, we can maintain muscle mass, keep our bones strong, and move well. The risk of falls decreases thanks to maintaining our mind-muscle connection. This is great news because falls are a major health factor as we age because we are less able to recover from serious injuries. Also, if you have children, you may notice they play on the floor a lot. I am sure you want to be able to play with the children in your family, and strength training allows us the opportunity to be strong enough to get down to and up from the floor safely. So, even though we may not be preparing to play a sport, strength training can prepare us for the things we want to be able to do in life.

While exercise has many tremendous benefits, it is not an excuse to eat poorly. You will never out exercise a poor diet. You do not need to "earn your Calories", and exercise certainly is not punishment for unhealthy choices. Let us treat exercise like the thing it is, a fun tool that can be used to help us reach our goals and age gracefully. Too much or too little can be detrimental to our health. We need to aim for the sweet spot where we get just enough.

Back to EPOC. EPOC stands for excess post-exercise oxygen consumption. I am sure you have heard of the "fat burning zone" of exercise that is the magic area where we burn more fat as an energy source. This is true. It happens, and if you are in the "fat burning zone", you will utilize fat as an energy source. However, exercising at a high intensity creates an oxygen debt within our cells. This occurs because the intensity we are working at is higher than the body can sustain on oxygen alone. So, it must use other sources to create ATP (adenosine triphosphate) to be used. Following exercise, the body must work harder over a longer period (i.e. burn more Calories) to return to the baseline levels of oxygen consumption. This process occurs during all levels of exercise intensity, but the oxygen deficit is greater, and therefore takes longer to return to baseline, during high intensity exercise. I am sure you have had the feeling where you just could not seem to catch your breath after a workout, that is EPOC at work. So, while we may burn fat in the fat burning zone, we get more return on our investment through strength training and interval style training than simply utilizing steady state cardio.

These benefits do not just apply to strength. If you need to build your aerobic capacity, you do not need to go out and run for a long period of time. If you do not actually enjoy going out running for hours on end or sitting on your cardio machine of choice, the good news is you do not have to. For conditioning, interval training has been shown to elicit similar physiological responses to steady state cardio. It is more time efficient, and a little less boring. If you do enjoy it, it is important to balance it with a smart strength training regimen and be mindful that you are not doing too much. This applies to competitive and recreational athletes.

When done properly, strength training is much more sustainable long term than running. It has plenty of health benefits to help you reach your goals too. Overall, the return on the investment of your time is much better spent in a smart strength training program. A good program gives you the ability to go run without issue but is built with the understanding the running is not the end-all-be-all when it comes to maintaining health.

If you are looking to find a good strength training program, and you decide not to use CH Health & Fitness, look for something that includes more than just strength training. We also need to be training our mobility and stability, and a good coach or trainer should also be helping you to cool down by getting you back into the parasympathetic state. It should not be random. It needs to be consistent enough for you to be able to see the progress you make, and then maybe add some variety every 3-6 weeks. It should not always be super high or super low intensity. It should have a mix of both, and some training right in the middle. It also needs to be a well thought out plan that considers your needs and history. Various reps and sets should be trained as well.

Remember that we do need some consistency in these areas so that we can see our progress. There should even be some aerobic based conditioning as well. Try to keep it low impact to avoid excess strain on the joints. We want to have balance so that we can move well under any circumstances. Please keep in mind that there are no mandatory exercises. There are patterns (squat, hinge, lunge, push, and pull are likely some you are most familiar with) that we do need to train, but exercises are just tools to train these patterns.

A good training strategy is to think like an athlete. This does not mean spending hours upon hours in the gym, and it does not mean doing overly intense exercises balancing on a bosu ball. What do athletes do differently? They train. They have specific goals and criteria they need to meet to be successful. Training is different from working out. It is not random. It is planned and executed with purposeful intention. They train in the weight room and within their respective arenas. The weight room becomes a place to improve mobility, power, speed, and strength. These are all important qualities to maintain as we age. The best athletes also know that the weight room is only a supporting tool. At a certain point, lifting more weight does not necessarily transfer to on field/court performance. So, they also spend hours mastering their crafts. The best athletes are masters of the fundamentals, and the fundamentals of their sport are not left out of their training. What does all of this practice lead to? A ton of movement outside of the weight room. For us, this looks like an increase in Non-Exercise Activity Thermogenesis (NEAT). It is important to be strong. It helps us reduce the chance of injury, is fun, and helps us to maintain the ability to be independent and do the things we want as we age. Plus, the right exercise program helps increase NEAT due to EPOC. But it is even more important to be active in all areas of our lives.

Even with all these benefits, exercise alone is not enough to help us reach our goals. Exercise really is not even the most important movement we get throughout the day either. The most important movement we get is NEAT. This is just a fancy way to think about all of the movement we do throughout the day which causes us to use up energy. This is why taking the stairs or parking further away can be a huge gamechanger. Think about it, if we exercise for one hour a day, that leaves 23 more hours. We will say that your habits are dialed in, and you are getting at least 8 hours of sleep per night. That leaves 15 more hours every single day. If we do not move, the exercise we do in that single hour is much less significant. We are designed to move. The simple act of going for a walk outdoors has been shown to increase productivity, increase energy levels, reduce symptoms of depression, improve self-esteem, and even improve physical traits like heart rate and blood pressure.

How can we increase our NEAT activities? Well that is up to you, but I can give you some strategies. One strategy is to set an alarm for every hour while at work and go for a walk each time it goes off. If you can, try to do so outside. If you cannot go for a walk outside, maybe go for one through the office, or maybe even just do some simple exercises like squats and pushups at your desk. You might look weird, but you will feel great. You can also create a rule like if you need to go upstairs, anything under 3 floors you will not use an elevator. When at work, the grocery store, or other venues, park further away so that you have to take extra steps to get where you are going. 10,000 steps per day by our hunter gatherer ancestors is actually a made-up number, but it is a great way to try to improve NEAT. Before shooting for this goal, measure your current steps per day, and create a smaller goal, and then build up to 10,000 steps per day. If you have a dog, dog walks are a tremendous way to get more steps in, and it is a great activity to do as a family. However, do not simply get a dog to increase your steps, dogs are a huge commitment. Make sure you are ready for the commitment of taking care of a dog. You can also just commit to family walks. I also encourage you to adopt and take away the power from inhumane breeders who use and abuse dogs. Adopting pets truly changes the lives of your pet and you. I know my life would not be the same if we had not adopted our dogs.

You may also want to pick up a hobby like gardening. Or anything that is going to get you on your feet and moving. There are so many options for increasing NEAT. Find out what works best in your situation. Even if your goals are weight gain, increasing NEAT is probably in your best interest for improving long term health. If you are an athlete, chances are you are moving plenty, and may not need to work as hard to get to 10,000 steps. Every situation is different, so allow your situation and goals to dictate how you implement this habit. Always remember that we cannot out train a bad diet.

Move

Now that you better understand why it is so important to move, we can get into how to implement the habit. The trick is to find what works best for you. We are all highly individual. I cannot tell you what is going to be best in your situation. That is something you must find on your own. A coach can help brainstorm ideas, but the execution falls on you. Use the notes section to brainstorm and track how different strategies work for you, and then work with your coach or accountability partner to really dial in what your best practice might be. Do not forget to continue the previous habits because they all work together. Focus on this habit for the next 4 weeks. Take more time if you need. Remember, we truly want this to become part of our lives.

- Take it Slow - Pick a single strategy to improve NEAT. Work to implement that strategy once a day. Use the notes section to notice how you feel and perform when you increase your activity.

- A Little More Challenging - Pick 2-3 strategies to improve NEAT. Work to implement those strategies into your day. Use the notes section to notice how you feel and perform when you increase your activity. Maybe start doing some research on specific exercise programs you want to get into.

- Ready for a Challenge - Implement strategies to improve your NEAT daily. Get to 10,000 steps a day. Exercise 3-4 times per week. Start to notice how exercise and increased levels of activity make you feel.

Notes

General notes about the habit:

How are you planning on implementing this habit?

How ready, willing, and able are you to implement your strategy? (for a reminder on how to use this activity, see page 28)

What are some potential roadblocks you may face?

What are some strategies you can use prepare for these roadblocks?

What have you noticed about how you feel, think, or act after implementing this habit?

Which Pillars do you feel that this habit impacts? Why?

Any questions, comments, or concerns to bring up with your coach?

References

Berardi, J., & Andrews, R. (2010). *The essentials of sport and exercise nutrition*. Precision Nutrition.

Boyle, M. (2004). *Functional training for sports* Human Kinetics Publishers.

Boyle, M. (2016). *New functional training for sports* Human Kinetics.

Bubbs, M. (2019). *Peak: The new science of athletic performance that is revolutionizing sports* Chelsea Green Publishing.

Connolly, F., & White, P. (2017). *Game changer* Simon and Schuster.

Craft, L. L., & Perna, F. M. (2004). The benefits of exercise for the clinically depressed. *Primary Care Companion to the Journal of Clinical Psychiatry, 6*(3), 104.

Gladwell, V. F., Brown, D. K., Wood, C., Sandercock, G. R., & Barton, J. L. (2013). The great outdoors: How a green exercise environment can benefit all. *Extreme Physiology & Medicine, 2*(1), 3.

Haff, G. G., & Triplett, N. T. (2015). *Essentials of strength training and conditioning 4th edition* Human kinetics.

Harari, Y. N. (2014). *Sapiens: A brief history of humankind* Random House.

Learney, P. (2014). *N1 nutritional programming: The fundamentals of nutritional programming.* ACA
Medina, J. (2011). *Brain rules: 12 principles for surviving and thriving at work, home, and school* ReadHowYouWant. Com.

Poliquin, Charles. *Poliquin Principles: Successful Methods for Strength and Mass Development.* Poliquin Performance Centers, 2006.

Rowan, A. E., Kueffner, T. E., & Stavrianeas, S. (2012). Short duration high-intensity interval training improves aerobic conditioning of female college soccer players. *International Journal of Exercise Science, 5*(3), 6.

Schjerve, I. E., Tyldum, G. A., Tjønna, A. E., Stølen, T., Loennechen, J. P., Hansen, H. E., Najjar, S. M. (2008). Both aerobic endurance and strength training programmes improve cardiovascular health in obese adults. *Clinical Science, 115*(9), 283-293.

Tsutsumi, T., Don, B. M., Zaichkowsky, L. D., & Delizonna, L. L. (1997). Physical fitness and psychological benefits of strength training in community dwelling older adults. *Applied Human Science, 16*(6), 257-266.

Verstegen, M., & Williams, P. (2014). *Every day is game day: Train like the pros with a no-holds-barred exercise and nutrition plan for peak performance* Penguin.

Walker, M. (2017). *Why we sleep: Unlocking the power of sleep and dreams* Simon and Schuster.

Habit 12: Live

You did it. You have gotten through all the habits. Congratulations! You have taken huge steps towards your goals. You are now equipped with the fundamental information that will help you to reach your goals. This last part really is not even a habit at all. This is a reminder. A reminder that life will happen. Do not get caught up in being perfect. None of us are perfect, and nobody expects you to be. Let me reiterate that. Nobody expects you to be perfect. So, do not expect yourself to be perfect. If a slip up happens, try to think of ways to learn from that experience, acknowledge that it happened and that there is nothing you can change because it is in the past, forgive yourself, and move on.

Remember that humans are social creatures. So, we must work to not create overbearing rules on our lives. Do not avoid an interaction with a friend or family member because they might want pizza for dinner. Pizza is delicious. Maybe even bring over some ice cream for dessert. This can serve as a break, a reminder that we are not going to be perfect, or a reminder of why you started this journey in the first place. It could very well be an opportunity to kick start a conversation with your friends and family on how they might start their own journey towards better health. However, never preach to them. When they are ready, they will seek you out. Until that moment, just be a good friend to them, and always offer your love and support. If it never happens, that is okay too. They are still the people we care about and will support no matter what.

So, I encourage you to have a night out with friends. Maybe even partake in some alcoholic drinks! You know the effects it might have on you, but the emotional benefit of going out could very well outweigh the physical repercussions. We evolved to cooperate and support each other, and we must never forget that. We feel better when we are with the right people. Plus, you have cultivated your circle of friends to be the supportive people you need in your life anyway. What was the point of doing that if you cannot go out and enjoy it? What is the point of making all this progress towards your goals if you cannot go to show people what you have accomplished and maybe even help them get closer to their goals? If you asked me, I would say that all our efforts might be wasted if we cannot share it with others.

The biggest steps we can take in any situation is to have a plan and execute that plan consistently over time. Perhaps, we know that hanging out with specific people means we are going to eat more food. Maybe a strategy is to practice time restricted eating and fasting until you see those friends. I cannot tell you what is going to work for each situation. But a good coach can help you brainstorm different ideas for tackling different situations. Experiment, track, and adjust. Just do not forget that we still need to be able to enjoy our time here on this magnificent planet.

References

Berardi, J., & Andrews, R. (2010). *The essentials of sport and exercise nutrition*. Precision Nutrition.

Harari, Y. N. (2014). *Sapiens: A brief history of humankind* Random House.

Sinek, S. (2014). *Leaders eat last: Why some teams pull together and others do not* Penguin.

187

Section V: The Next Level

You have taken tremendous steps towards optimizing your health. Awesome work! You should be proud of the hard work you have put in. I also want to provide some information on things we can do to truly take our health and performance to the next level. This section will hit on things such as supplements, eating at restaurants, meditation, an introduction to functional medicine, further readings, and will be wrapped up with some final thoughts and key takeaways.

These chapters will be quick. They are here to wet your whistle and pique your interest. Each of them could be (and are) books of their own. There will be no habits within this section. It is purely informational. However, remember the premise of this whole book: experiment with different things to find what works best for you in your situation.

Supplements

Supplements have become vastly popular. This section will serve as an introduction to supplements. There are so many out there that to be able to touch on them all would be an entire book. Remember, we want to keep it simple.

The baseline of our health should always come from whole food sources. However, if supplements are a bridge to help you kick start your journey into health, I am all for it.

Before we even get into it, we should remember that the quality of anything we put into our bodies plays a role in how these things interact within our bodies. To ensure you are getting what you are paying for, it is important to use supplements that use quality ingredients. 2 that I go to for my own personal supplements are Thorne (www.thorne.com) and Momentous (www.livemomentous.com). You don't have to use them, but should you choose to head to https://coreyhobbs.com/blog/f/supplements-101 to take advantage of the discounted prices. Full disclosure, I do receive a small percentage of anything you purchase if you use any of the links there. Currently, I do not have the opportunity to offer a discount on Momentous, but I assure you they are worth the price. These are just 2 of the many companies out there that do the right thing. They do not use fillers or additives and have the health of their clients as their top priority.

Should you choose another brand of supplement you should look for the NSF Certified for Sport seal. This ensures that the product was tested and contains what it says it does. 3rd party testing is in our best interest as consumers to ensure that we are getting the things we are paying for. This also means that our products will not be contaminated with illegal substances should you be an individual that has to succumb to drug testing. Always make sure to verify with the governing agency of items you will be drug tested for.
First, we will start with some baseline supplements that would be benefitted by nearly everyone.

The Essentials

Multi-Vitamin

The nutrients in our food are not as high as they once were. The reason for this is that the way we farm today actually depletes the nutrients from the soil. The soil is then never given an opportunity to replenish its nutrients from insects, or grazing animals. So, the first place we want to start is with a quality multi-vitamin. It should contain all the essential vitamins and minerals in adequate amounts.

Magnesium

Magnesium is responsible for over 300 processes in our body. The more we learn about the body, that number seems to keep growing. It takes part in muscle contractions, improves sleep, improves insulin sensitivity, improves metabolic function, and helps with bowel movements to name only a small percentage of the things it does in the body. Most people are deficient in magnesium as well. With as many processes as it is involved in, it is important we work to give our bodies what it needs. Aim for 600-1,000 mg per day.

Fish Oil

Fish oil (or Omega-3 Fats) is responsible for healthy cardiovascular and nervous systems, improving insulin sensitivity, and immune function. We learned earlier that we need to work to get our omega-3:omega-6 ratio close to 1:2 or 1:3, and a supplement can help us do that. This is especially true if you are not someone who enjoys eating fatty fish. Shoot for 2-6 grams per day.

Vitamin D3

Vitamin D is important to maintain healthy bones, a healthy immune system, and has anti-depressive benefits. Vitamin D can be a bit tricky. The wrong kind, and we might not get the benefits. Ideally, we would get ample sunlight to ensure we are getting enough of it. Before supplementing, I suggest spending as much time in direct sunlight with as much skin exposed as possible. Do not stay out long enough to burn. That should be our first choice in trying to improve Vitamin D levels. In the winter when we spend less time outside, or if you're in an environment where the sun is not out for very long, such as Alaska, it is a good idea to supplement with Vitamin D3 and K2 as they work well together. 1,000 - 2,000 IU is a good place to start.

Next, we will discuss supplements for performance. These can be used in addition to the basics.

Supplements for Performance

Creatine

Creatine has long been thought of as a meathead supplement that only has one purpose: to make people bigger. However, it is one of the most well researched supplements with benefits ranging from performance and strength all the way to improved cognitive function as well as healing and protecting from traumatic brain injury. With the many benefits of creatine, I debated putting it in the category for everyone. But, since we want to focus on the basics in this book, I kept it in this section. Just know that most people could probably benefit from creatine supplementation. Despite what you may have heard, there is no real need for a "loading" period. Simply take 5g per day.

Protein

We learned that our bodies use amino acids from our amino acid pool to help repair damaged tissues. So, a good way to ensure our pools are filled is to ensure those pools are filled. There are a few ways to do this. You can use an Essential Amino Acid (EAA) supplement, you can use a protein powder, or a plant based protein powder. If you go the route of protein powders, I suggest whey protein from grass-fed cows. If you elect for plant protein, ensure it uses quality sourced ingredients and has all of the essential amino acids. Momentous makes great plant based and grass-fed whey products. I like to switch between the two. The evidence for the "anabolic window" seems to be pointing toward the idea that there is not really one. However, it is simple to ingest a powder right after exercise. This way you it is simple to get enough throughout the day. Shoot for about 20-25g of protein per meal. If your goal is gaining weight, you may want to experiment with adding carbohydrates to your post training shake as well.

Caffeine

Caffeine has been shown to help with both endurance and strength athletes. It has been used to boost performance for a long time. When using caffeine, start with smaller doses, and work up if you need to in order to find your optimal dose. 2 mg/kg of bodyweight is a good place to start. Do not use it too late in the afternoon as it will negatively impact sleep and recovery. Also, use coffee or a tablet. When taken in energy drinks or pre-workout supplements there are a lot of added things in there we do not really need. Not to mention you run the risk of failing a drug test if the pre-workout is not NSF certified. The feeling pre-workouts give us usually comes from beta alanine anyway. And it is much more cost effective to buy them separately. Speaking of beta alanine...

<u>Beta Alanine</u>

Beta Alanine works better for endurance athletes, but many strength athletes like it for the tingly sensation it gives them. It acts as an acidic buffer in the cells which is why it is better for performance over a long period of time as opposed to short, intense bursts of output. Start small with beta alanine as the tingling sensation can become quite distracting. This is especially true if you have never used it before. Start with about 2-3g.

Pre-Pregnancy, Pregnancy, and Breastfeeding

If you are thinking of becoming pregnant, are pregnant, or are breastfeeding, there are some supplements that have been shown to benefit you and your baby. Speak with your doctor before adding a new supplement.

<u>Prenatal Vitamins</u>

Prenatal vitamins are basically multivitamins with extra folate. Folate is critical for the development of the fetus and baby. However, we should be careful that we are getting folate not folic acid. Folic acid blocks the uptake of folate within our bodies (a pretty big issue when we consider the fact that most processed foods are "fortified" with folic acid). The active version of folate is often listed as 5-MTHF (Methyl tetrahydrofolate if you were wondering).

<u>Phospholipids</u>

In addition to fish oil, phospholipids, such as phosphatidylcholine and phosphatidylserine, are other fatty acids that are essential for development. Choline is essential for nerve and brain function. Plus, phospholipids make up our cell walls. Which is extra important if you are a baby or fetus and growing constantly. Phosphatidylserine - 100mg 1-3 times per day. Phosphatidylcholine - about 900mg a day

Recovering from Injury

When recovering from injury, we want to limit inflammation. We do not want to eliminate it completely. Inflammation is a natural part of the healing process. Limit pain relievers. They are good for relieving pain in the short term but can hinder the healing process long term. Make sure to eat plenty of food so that the body has enough nutrients that it needs to complete the repair process. Ensure you are getting plenty of healthy fats and limit the amount of processed carbohydrates per day. Curcumin, garlic, berries, and green tea (both in supplement and tea form) also can help during this period.

This is by no means an all-inclusive list of supplements or situations where supplements might help. Make sure you are getting supplements that contain the things they say they do. Remember food should be our first choice for nutrients. Supplements are a tool to supplement our diets. They are not there to justify eating poorly, and they are not to be some magical experience that all the sudden makes your goals and dreams come true. For information on supplements, I highly recommend examine.com. They do not take donations and objectively examine all the information on supplements that is currently available.

References

Andres, R. H., Ducray, A. D., Schlattner, U., Wallimann, T., & Widmer, H. R. (2008). Functions and effects of creatine in the central nervous system. *Brain Research Bulletin, 76*(4), 329-343.

Berardi, J., & Andrews, R. (2010). *The essentials of sport and exercise nutrition.* Precision Nutrition.

Bubbs, M. (2019). *Peak: The new science of athletic performance that is revolutionizing sports* Chelsea Green Publishing.

Gualano, B., Artioli, G. G., Poortmans, J. R., & Junior, A. H. L. (2010). Exploring the therapeutic role of creatine supplementation. *Amino Acids, 38*(1), 31-44.

Haff, G. G., & Triplett, N. T. (2015). *Essentials of strength training and conditioning 4th edition* Human kinetics.

Hyman, M. (2018). *Food: What the heck should I eat?* Hachette UK.

LaValle, J. B. (2013). *Your blood never lies: How to read a blood test for a longer, healthier life* Square One Publishers, Inc.

LaValle, J. B., & Yale, S. L. (2004). *Cracking the metabolic code: The nine keys to peak health* Basic Health Publications, Inc.

Ross, R. G., Hunter, S. K., Hoffman, M. C., McCarthy, L., Chambers, B. M., Law, A. J., Freedman, R. (2015). Perinatal phosphatidylcholine supplementation and early childhood behavior problems: Evidence for CHRNA7 moderation. *American Journal of Psychiatry, 173*(5), 509-516.

Sakellaris, G., Kotsiou, M., Tamiolaki, M., Kalostos, G., Tsapaki, E., Spanaki, M., Evangeliou, A. (2006). Prevention of complications related to traumatic brain injury in children and adolescents with creatine administration: An open label randomized pilot study. *Journal of Trauma and Acute Care Surgery, 61*(2), 322-329.

Sullivan, P. G., Geiger, J. D., Mattson, M. P., & Scheff, S. W. (2000). Dietary supplement creatine protects against traumatic brain injury. *Annals of Neurology, 48*(5), 723-729.

Tarnopolsky, M. A., & Beal, M. F. (2001). Potential for creatine and other therapies targeting cellular energy dysfunction in neurological disorders. *Annals of Neurology, 49*(5), 561-574.

Verstegen, M., & Williams, P. (2014). *Every day is game day: Train like the pros with a no-holds-barred exercise and nutrition plan for peak performance* Penguin.

Walker, M. (2017). *Why we sleep: Unlocking the power of sleep and dreams* Simon and Schuster.

Avoiding Toxins

Although the title may have you believe that this section is all about detoxifying which leads you to believe you should go grab your favorite detox tea, it is not. With all the habits presented here, chances are that our bodies have the tools necessary to clear most toxins. At this stage, we are likely 90% there.

Let us get the obvious out of the way. If you are smoking cigarettes or drinking alcohol in excess, you are loading your body full of toxins. By increasing the body's toxic load there is simply no way you are going to cultivate health. If your goal is truly optimizing health and improving the Pillars of Health, these are not things we need in our lives. If you struggle with these, utilize the same approach we used throughout this book – start small and work until you have reached your goal.

I mentioned earlier that sleep is a huge part of the detoxifying process. Well, sweat is too which is why saunas and exercise are excellent detox tools. Going to the bathroom is another way we detox. When we give our bodies the nutrients they need, they can clear toxins rather effectively. Unfortunately, even when we get everything right, an overabundance of toxins in our systems can lead to issues with sleep, messed up hormones, and an inability to lose fat. What this section is about is one of the best ways to detox our systems that often goes unmentioned, and you may have already guessed it by the title – avoiding toxins altogether.

Unfortunately, toxins are present in many convenience products offered today. Worse yet, they are present in some unexpected places as well. We already talked about the importance of filtering our water and switching to glass food storage options. So, what are some other places that we should be wary of toxins?

Let us start with cosmetic products. For many of us, these are products that we use daily. Here is a short list: toothpaste, deodorant, shampoo, conditioner, shaving cream, face wash, lotion, and makeup. Okay, maybe it is not very short. The fact is, there are a ton of household products out there can wreak havoc on our bodies and all its systems. BPA and all its cousins, phthalates, parabens, and microplastics to name a handful. These examples specifically mimic estrogen, and this means that they bind to estrogen receptors in our bodies which then changes the way estrogen works. Even if you are a male, this is not a good thing. Males need proper amounts of estrogen too, and without it, things can go awry. It could be the reason that last little bit of belly fat just will not budge.

Now for some not so obvious places. For one, many furniture pieces, home décor, construction materials, and even electronics create toxic gases that we breathe in daily. To make matters worse, many cleaning products and pesticides do the same. We basically create our own toxic world inside our homes. This leads to increased risks of cancer and other issues, and if children are present, they are at greater risks. The issue is not only the hormonal implications, but toxins have been shown to impact our genes causing potentially dangerous mutations. This cascading effect can lead to sickness and disease, and we may not even realize that it is happening.

Chemicals such as naphtha, benzene, petroleum distillates, butoxyethanol, and propylene glycol are all found in many popular house cleaners. These are all known or suspected carcinogenic substances. Furniture and electronics often formaldehyde and fire retardant as well. A new home is going to have these in even larger quantities due to the materials being brand new and likely exposed to chemicals more recently.

Pesticides and herbicides are also highly toxic, and we should be avoiding them. There is a reason Monsanto recently lost a lawsuit that will cost them billions of dollars. These things work because they target the nervous system of whatever it is they promise to kill. Do you want to know what they impact in humans? The same thing. They work have a huge impact on our nervous systems, and we would be best off if we simply avoided these all together.

Clearly, this paints a rather dire picture. But there is certainly hope. We have talked previously about ways to reduce toxic exposure in our water, food containers, and cookware. There are plenty of strategies that we can utilize in our homes as well!

One of the easiest strategies for ridding toxic gases within our homes is opening the windows. Just a few minutes a day goes a long way, but you may find it so refreshing that you opt to do it longer. There is a reason opening windows and letting fresh air in is so refreshing – it allows the toxins to clear out of our homes. You can also get a HEPA air purifier. These do an excellent job of cleaning up our air, but they can be a little pricey.

Then we need to work to start avoiding all the toxins found in other areas. One major area we can start to improve right away is minimizing plastic use. This has a benefit that is twofold. For one, it is better for us because we do not ingest (yes this happens on the micro level when we use these products) any plastics. Two, single use plastics are huge burden on the environment. Even our organic produce in plastic containers could cause potential issues. They take a long time do degrade, and they only get smaller which causes problem with our ocean life. By minimizing or removing these entirely, we are not only being conscious of our own health, but the health of the environment as well.

Now for the cosmetic and cleaning products. This can be very challenging. Fortunately, companies are starting to realize the harmful effects of many toxins, and people are too which means they are demanding higher quality products from those companies. Our purchasing habits can be a powerful tool to elicit change. Look for products that are free of phthalates, parabens, fragrances, dyes, plastics, and even trace amounts of metals like aluminum (looking at you, deodorant).

Most of those are obvious. However, fragrances (and this is true for flavor in foods too) is a pretty broad term. There is little regulation for what goes into fragrances and flavors. So, a company merely argues that a product (or toxin) is essential to the fragrance or flavor, and they have a large amount of freedom of what they can include

What is another product containing BPA you handle almost every day and is likely letting BPA in your system? Receipts. They are everywhere, and every purchase comes with one. We touch it, and the BPA gets into our systems from our skin. What are we to do? We could simply ask not to receive receipts. But many stores are allowing for email receipts. We still get our receipt, and our skin stays BPA free.

Avoiding toxins in our everyday products is challenging. This is one area which I struggle with the most. Food is easy. We stick to whole foods and it is hard to go wrong. Fortunately, there are some good companies that are working to create safe products. Even better for us is that the Environmental Working Group (EWG) has an app that lets you scan products to know for sure. You can find it in your phone's app store. Simply scan the barcode and it gives a score based on the quality of that product and its ingredients. It does not have every product out there. But it does have a lot. If it does not have a product you scan, it gives the option of submitting a picture of the product and its ingredients. This is not a guarantee the product will get reviewed, but it does improve the likelihood. Head to https://www.ewg.org for more information on products with contaminants and loads of other information on how to stay healthy. I love having the EWG app and website as quick references if there is ever a product I may not sure about. I highly recommend utilizing this free tool.

One last note, there are situations in which a real detox like chelation therapy is needed. If you believe you have been exposed to significant amounts of toxic mold, heavy metals, or pesticides you should work with a functional medicine practitioner to find out if this is something you may need. The treatments can be dangerous without professional help, so make sure you are working with someone who knows what they are doing!

References

Asprey, D. (2018). *Game changers: What leaders, innovators, and mavericks do to win at life* HarperCollins.

Asprey, D. (2020). *Superhuman: A bulletproof guide to age backwards and maybe even live forever.* HarperCollins

Hyman, M. (2018). *Food: What the heck should I eat?* Hachette UK.

Hyman, M. (2020). *Food Fix: How to Save Our Health, Our Economy, Our Communities, and Our Planet -- One Bite at a Time.* Little, Brown Spark

Kresser, C. (2017). *Unconventional medicine: Join the revolution to reinvent healthcare, reverse chronic disease, and create a practice you love* Lioncrest Publishing.

LaValle, J. B. (2013). *Your blood never lies: How to read a blood test for a longer, healthier life* Square One Publishers, Inc.

LaValle, J. B., & Yale, S. L. (2004). *Cracking the metabolic code: The nine keys to peak health* Basic Health Publications, Inc

Lynch, B. (2018). *Dirty genes* Harper One, New York.

Perlmutter, D. (2018). *Grain brain: The surprising truth about wheat, carbs, and sugar--your brain's silent killers* Hachette UK.

Tackling Restaurants

I do not expect you to never go out. I told you in the last habit that we still need to live. So, what should we do when we go out to eat? The good news is that there are restaurants out there that do use the quality ingredients you learned about. Try to find those places. They are usually pretty good at letting people know where their ingredients come from.

What happens when you cannot find a place like this? Well you already have the tools you need. You know what to look out for. Now you just put it to use. There are almost always healthy options at restaurants. We just need to look out for the ones that are not actually so healthy for us. Things that are cooked in or with hydrogenated oils we know we want to avoid. We should avoid industrial meat, and we should focus on whole foods. Be careful with salad dressings and other toppings. These tend to be a big place that added sugar and other additives hideout. However, for the most part, our same baseline principles apply in restaurants. We can also ask what is in certain meals along with the ingredients used to prepare the food. This way we understand exactly what we are getting. Plus, it could serve as an opportunity to give an understanding of why you chose to be healthy to the people you go out with. Do not preach at them, but they might ask why you choose a salad as opposed to your regular burger. Explain your reasoning, and if they want more information, they will come to you. When we give information to those who are not ready for it, the information often goes ignored anyway. We cannot force change on people who are not ready to start down the path of change.

But we can also just enjoy food from restaurants sometimes. We should not live in fear of going out to eat, and we cannot live life in a bubble. It alienates us from the people we want to spend time with. We should always strive to be healthy but indulging occasionally likely will not send you off the deep end. When we do indulge, we often feel bad, and that is both because of the lesser quality foods and sometimes a little bit of guilt. That is okay though. We knew we were not always going to be perfect going into this. It can serve as a reminder of why we utilize these habits the way we do.

So how should you tackle eating out? It really depends. What is your goal right now? Do you eat out often? Is this a special event that you do not always get the opportunity to attend? If you are already eating out a good amount, try to make healthier choices. If you are in a situation where you do not eat out a lot, and it is a special occasion, maybe let the rules slide a little bit for that occasion. There is no black and white. Health happens on a continuum, and where we are on that continuum is a result of our goals and habits leading up to that time. If you have been struggling with your habits, maybe focus on whole foods. Or maybe you don't, but use it as an opportunity to remind yourself why you started down this path in the first place. It is okay to go off the rails sometimes. We have all done it. Sometimes you blink and that whole pizza or pint of Ben and Jerry's has vanished. Use these types of events as learning opportunities and understand that another opportunity to make a choice more in tune with your goals is right around the corner. Be kind to yourself and move on.

References

Berardi, J., & Andrews, R. (2010). *The essentials of sport and exercise nutrition*. Precision Nutrition.

Bubbs, M. (2019). *Peak: The new science of athletic performance that is revolutionizing sports* Chelsea Green Publishing.

Learney, P. (2014). *N1 nutritional programming: The fundamentals of nutritional programming*. ACA

Meditation

I would be doing the Psychology Pillar a huge disservice if I did not mention meditation. Meditation is now becoming more popular and mainstream. This is great because there are a ton of positive benefits to it. It is also likely that meditation is not as odd as what you are picturing. We do not have to sit quietly on a pillow with our legs folded and chanting to ourselves. That can be a form of meditation, but it is not the only way. There are also plenty of tools out there that can help us start to put meditation to good use.

What exactly is meditation then? Meditation can really be boiled down to the simple act of being in the present moment. You can be aware of the things going on around you, but the only thing that matters is the current moment. Believe it or not, the breathing exercise we did all the way back in the beginning of the book is a form of meditation.

You might still be on the fence about giving it a try, so, let us talk about some of the benefits that meditation can bring before we get into how to do it. These are all researched benefits, and things that I have experienced firsthand. I was on the fence for a long time about meditation, and now it is something I make sure to take the time to do in my day.

One of the biggest benefits is improved sleep. We learned about how critical sleep is for our health, and meditation is a great way to positively impact sleep. Not just sleep either, it has been shown to increase deep sleep which is important because that is the most restorative portion of our sleep. This happens because meditation is an excellent tool to get into that parasympathetic (rest and digest) state. By allowing ourselves to focus only in the moment, the stressors of the past and future no longer have a hold on us. This allows our bodies to return from their overstressed state to an environment more conducive for rest. Meditation can even be as restorative as taking a nap in the afternoon without the groggy feeling when we wake up. It has less time cost, and you finish feeling refreshed and ready to tackle the rest of the day.

We can also improve our relationships. Through the process of meditation, we can become more aware of our thoughts and responses to those thoughts. With consistent meditation, we are less reactive because we can recognize the feelings growing inside of us. We are then able to respond in more constructive ways and have meaningful conversations without anger or anxiety. Not only has it been shown to improve relationships with others, but also our relationship with ourselves. Remember that we are the number one person we spend time with. Meditation has been shown to improve the overall sense of well-being of individuals with regular practice.

Do you know what neuroplasticity is? If not, that is okay. It is basically the rewiring that occurs within our brains. Our brains are highly adaptable, and when given the proper stimuli, they can improve for the better. Our brains do not have to get worse as we age! This means that we can improve brain function, and productivity through the practice of meditation. Seems like a pretty good thing to me.

The list goes on and on of the benefits attributed to meditation. Reduced symptoms of depression and anxiety, reduced effects of aging, improved eyesight, improved self-control, improved fertility, reduced frequency and intensity of migraines, reduced symptoms of ADD and ADHD, and even better sex. That is right, meditation can help us have better sex. By practicing being present in the moment, we can decrease the stress hormones within our bodies and perform at our absolute best.

Are you on board with meditation now? If not, that is your prerogative. I still encourage you to try it out. What is the worst that can happen? It only takes a few minutes, and the potential benefits far outweigh the time cost. In fact, more and more doctors are beginning to see the positive benefits and incorporate it not only in their own lives, but the lives of their patients as well. It is even being utilized by high performers such as professional athletes.

How do we do it? Start small. As with anything, it is important to not bite off more than we can chew. Start with a couple minutes, and slowly build up. There is also the idea of clearing your mind. This is impossible. Your mind does not turn off. Allow thoughts to come and go. Simply notice them, but do not act on them. Let them naturally flow in and out of your mind. A great place to start is with the breathing exercise from earlier, and now simply count your breaths. Count to 10, and then start over or go backwards. If you lose count, start back at 1. Do not worry about thoughts coming and going. Just try to be present with your breath. Set a timer for however long you would like to go, and then go until the timer goes off. It really can be that easy. If you have pain anywhere in the process, notice it. But just notice that you have discomfort in an area. Instead of "my back hurts", simply note that there is discomfort in your back. This allows you to remove the focus of attention from your pain. The more you practice this, the more discomfort will likely decrease. The best part of meditation is that there are so many ways to add it to our lives! A walk in nature, yoga, or even simple breathing exercises are all forms of meditation. Each of them works to keep you present in the moment. Experiment with different kinds and find what works for you in your unique situation.

What if you are not ready to try it on your own? I was not there right away either. Luckily, there are apps like Headspace and Ten Percent Happier that have guided sessions to help you along the way. I got my start with Headspace's free version, and even upgraded to the paid version when I started noticing all the positive benefits. This book might not even exist if it were not for meditation (hopefully that is a good thing)! Now I can meditate on my own, but it is still refreshing to participate in guided meditations to rehash some of the skills.

There are also numerous books, courses, and retreats should you decide you really want to dive in on meditation. But I do suggest starting small and working to more advanced methods like those I just mentioned. Take 5-10 minutes a day to meditate and start reaping the numerous positive benefits within your life.

If you were looking for a single tool to enhance all four Pillars of Health, meditation would be it. It may be the closest thing we have to a "magic pill", and it is completely free.

References

Berardi, J., & Andrews, R. (2010). *The essentials of sport and exercise nutrition.* Precision Nutrition.

Bubbs, M. (2019). *Peak: The new science of athletic performance that is revolutionizing sports* Chelsea Green Publishing.

Davis, D. M., & Hayes, J. A. (2011). What are the benefits of mindfulness? A practice review of psychotherapy-related research. *Psychotherapy, 48*(2), 198.

Fletcher, E. (2019). *Stress less, accomplish more: Meditation for busy minds* Boxtree.

Horowitz, S. (2010). Health benefits of meditation: What the newest research shows. *Alternative and Complementary Therapies, 16*(4), 223-228.

https://www.headspace.com/science/meditation-benefits

https://www.tenpercent.com/

Hyman, M. (2018). *Food: What the heck should I eat?* Hachette UK.

LaValle, J. B., & Yale, S. L. (2004). *Cracking the metabolic code: The nine keys to peak health* Basic Health Publications, Inc.

Schreiner, I., & Malcolm, J. P. (2008). The benefits of mindfulness meditation: Changes in emotional states of depression, anxiety, and stress. *Behaviour Change, 25*(3), 156-168.

Shonin, E., Van Gordon, W., & Griffiths, M. D. (2013). Meditation as medication: Are attitudes changing? *Br J Gen Pract, 63*(617), 654.

An Introduction to Functional Medicine

Functional medicine is another item that is now becoming more mainstream. With athletes and celebrities alike using the positive benefits to optimize their health and performance. There is a good reason for this too: it works. Before we get into what functional medicine is, we need to understand why western medicine and our current system of healthcare is not designed to keep us healthy.

Western medicine will certainly keep us alive. There is no denying that. If we are dying, in a car accident, need a limb reattached, or need an operation, you bet we want to be in a hospital that specializes in keeping us alive. The current system is great for acute injury or illness but struggles in keeping people healthy long term. It is very responsive instead of being proactive or preventative.

For acute events such as these, western medicine flourishes. Unfortunately, events such as these are not the biggest threats to our health we face in this age. Chronic diseases such as diabetes, obesity, heart disease, and neurological conditions which all are made worse by inflammation and the standard American diet are the biggest threats to our longevity we face today. We are great at prolonging life, but not necessarily quality of life in tandem.

There are many reasons that this happens, but the bottom line is that the system is not currently set up to create an environment in which healthy people become our priority. Did you know that to become a doctor, there is very little to no nutritional training required? If you have taken anything from this book, I hope that the idea of nutrition being a key component to unlocking health is on that list. Recall your last doctor's appointment. It probably went something like this: Check in and wait in the waiting room for 30-45 minutes. Then you get checked out by a nurse who takes down your symptoms. Then you wait some more for the doctor to come in. Once the doctor is in, he likely went over your symptoms, did some general checks, gave you a prescription or a suggestion for over the counter drugs, and left. On average, doctors are only able to spend about 15 minutes with their patients, and patients are shuffled in and out consistently throughout the day. If that example above was not your last doctor's visit, consider yourself lucky.

Due to the short amount of time doctors spend with patients, they are not always able to truly get to know their patients. Unfortunately, we become a list of symptoms that he must fix, and fixing the symptoms usually entails a prescription. This prescription likely includes a host of its own side effects that might even require another prescription to address the side effects down the line. Eventually, we are taking more pills than we can count, and we do not even feel any better.

Blame is often placed on our genes for many of our health issues. Our genes are death sentences that can never be changed, and we are doomed to a life of disease and unhappiness. I can recall a point in time when I was much younger where my dad lost a good amount of weight, and my sister noted that she cannot blame any weight gain on him anymore. In her mind, our dad's genes directly influenced her, and she was not in control. Is this really the case? Fortunately, it is not. In the book *Dirty Genes,* Dr. Ben Lynch lays out some pretty easy steps on how we can influence our genes. He states, "Contrary to what so many scientists and doctors believe, our genetic destiny isn't fixed. It can be edited, rewritten, changed. We just need to know how." He then continues that "we can transform our genetic destiny through a combination of diet, supplements, sleep, stress relief, and reduced exposure to environmental toxins (the toxins in our food, water, air, and products)." Go back and re-read that last sentence. The tools to rewrite our genes are in the habits that we have gone through within this book. This is not something I just believe, but it is also supported by epigenetic research. Epigenetics is the idea that environmental factors, such as nutrition and physical environment, play critical roles in shaping how our genes impact us, and how we can manipulate these factors in order to produce different results. Gone are the days where we can blame our relatives for our poor genetics. The power is in our hands.

To add to the issue is that we see a plethora of specialists within the medical field. Specializing is not a problem by itself. However, it is a problem if the only lens that a problem is viewed from is that specialized lens. For example, a GI specialist might look at your stomach issues, but not suggest a nutritional change because that is not part of their expertise. Or a brain specialist might examine your head, but not understand that much of our neurotransmitters come from our gut. As we have learned, proper nutrition can impact every system within our bodies, but nutrition is a topic barely covered, if at all, within the medicinal curriculums. We need a system in which it is understood that what happens in one area of the body, or our lives, can have significant ramifications in almost every other area of our lives. Our bodies are not a conglomeration of individual systems. They are intricate networks of systems which interact and work closely together, and they are constantly working to heal themselves. We just need to give them the tools necessary to do so.

The good news is that we are starting to see a shift. The shift is not only in how we view and understand our genes, but also how we view and understand individual patients and the issues that they have. The main idea behind functional medicine is that each individual that comes in is just that, an individual. Not a list of symptoms, but a unique blend of environment and circumstance that has brought that person to the current status of health. The practitioner and the patient then work together to create a sustainable plan that does not just treat symptoms. Instead, the plan works to get to the root of why disease has come around in the first place. This plan not only details medicinal treatments, but emotional, nutritional, and lifestyle treatments as well. It is truly a holistic approach to our health. Sessions with functional medicine practitioners last longer than 15 minutes, and practitioners work to; know and understand patients. The shift is gradual, but it is headed in the correct direction. In 2016, the Cleveland Clinic opened the Center for Functional Medicine led by Dr. Mark Hyman. Dr. Hyman went on to found the Ultra Wellness Center. Within these centers, western medicine and functional medicine work hand in hand to get to the root of problems for each patient. Dr. Hyman is not going at it alone either. There are several tremendous functional medicine practitioners around the globe working to change the status quo of medicine. The current status quo is not the fault of the doctors either. The current system is set up in such a way that doctors need to follow this path to make a living. In fact, doctors are some of the most stressed out and overworked individuals within society. We need a system that benefits the doctors we work with as much as we do for us as patients.

As you can see, western and functional medicine can and should work together to get to the root of problems. So, this section is by no means a suggestion that you stop seeing your doctor. Instead, consider working with a functional medicine practitioner (head to https://www.ifm.org/find-a-practitioner/ if you're interested) in conjunction with your regular doctor.

Functional medicine is not currently covered by many insurance providers. So, it can be quite costly. While it is an investment in your health, you may not be able to commit to something like that right now. What should you do if that is the case? There are a variety of books designed to give you control of your health. They will be listed in the further reading section, but I will go over 2 of them here as well. *Your Blood Never Lies* goes over how to read your blood test, and it gives the ranges for optimal health we should aim for. This book also details lifestyle tips and supplements that can help should we need it. *Dirty Genes* chronicles the steps we can take to take control of our genes to make them work for us instead of against us.

If you have an issue that has plagued you for a long time, and you cannot quite get to the cause, it could be time to investigate functional medicine. If everything feels fine, and your lab results are typically normal, use the books above to dive into your health. It might also be a good idea to meet with a functional medicine practitioner just to ensure everything is great under the hood. We need western medicine, and we would be a mess without its ability to respond to acute, traumatic events. However, we need the mentality of functional medicine in getting to the root causes of issues as opposed to treating a list of symptoms. There are even places like The Ultra Wellness Center that does an excellent job of marrying Western and Functional medicine practices. I think we have only seen the tip of the iceberg here, and places like this will begin to become more and more mainstream. We are as unique inside as we are outside, and there is no cookie cutter approach that can be applied to improve every person's health.

I believe in this approach so much that I plan on becoming a functional medicine practitioner in the future, and it is why I work to tailor my approach to the needs of everyone I work with. I do not believe in one size fits all prescriptions, and you should not either.

References

Hyman, M. (2018). *Food: What the heck should I eat?* Hachette UK.

Jones, D. S., Bland, J. S., & Quinn, S. (2005). What is functional medicine. *Textbook of Functional Medicine,* 5-14.

Kresser, C. (2017). *Unconventional medicine: Join the revolution to reinvent healthcare, reverse chronic disease, and create a practice you love* Lioncrest Publishing.

Kumar, S. (2016). Burnout and doctors: Prevalence, prevention and intervention. Paper presented at the *Healthcare, 4*(3) 37.

LaValle, J. B. (2013). *Your blood never lies: How to read a blood test for a longer, healthier life* Square One Publishers, Inc.

Lynch, B. (2018). *Dirty genes* Harper One, New York.

Perlmutter, D. (2018). *Grain brain: The surprising truth about wheat, carbs, and sugar--your brain's silent killers* Hachette UK.

Shanahan, C. (2016). *Deep Nutrition: Why Your Genes Need Traditional Food.* Flatiron Books

Zaidi, F. B. A. (2019). Organizational role stress and job burnout among doctors. *Omegademy Journal of Psychological Research, 1*(1), 13-26.

Closing Thoughts and Further Readings

Thank you for allowing me to help you along your journey towards health. By now, you should have a sound understanding of lifelong habits that can help you keep the Pillars of Health strong. I truly hope that you found the information within this book to be easy to digest and helpful. Remember that change is not instant. Instead, it is constant. I still work to master these baseline habits every single day, and I am nowhere near perfect. Do not expect perfection. Expect improvement. Every day is an opportunity to get closer to your goals. If you're looking for a coach for performance, nutrition, or even just life, head to https://www.coreyhobbss.com. My sole purpose is to help you reach your goals once I am your coach.

You will notice that there is no mention of severe Calorie restriction, fad diets, counting Calories, or weighing food. These often consume a lot of time and end up being an additional stressor within our lives. We already talked about the need to reduce stress in our lives. So, using a method like this is not worth the extra time and stress in my opinion. By focusing on quality, whole foods and tuning into our bodies, we are much more likely to reach our goals. We are also less likely to have a big rebound effect those other methods often come with. The bottom line is that we want to keep things simple and stress free. These baseline habits are more than enough to help you reach your goals regardless of where you start. Remember that we are looking for long term health, and we are not looking for quick solutions no matter how tempting they might be. When in doubt, ask yourself if a decision will positively or negatively impact any of the Pillars. This is a simple heuristic that could keep the guesswork out of your healthy decision-making process.

We talked briefly on how the current system is not designed with our health in mind. Is there anything we can do about it? We can. Every trip to the supermarket we have the option of voting with our dollars. We can either buy the foods of the standard American diet that will continue the status quo that is making us more sick, or we can choose to purchase healthy foods and force companies and the government to put systems in place that align with health instead of profits. We have more power than we think we do. We need to exercise that power any chance we get. You could also write or call your local, state, and federal representatives to ensure that they understand that we need to be prioritizing our health and so that they do not lay over and allow big corporations to call the shots when it comes to our health and nutrition.

Health is the base of the pyramid when it comes to our lives. Without it, we cannot perform in the way we want to in any domain. If we want to master the field, the boardroom, the studio, or any other area, we must first prioritize our health. When we prioritize our health and well-being, performance follows. We are even learning that our health could influence the health of our ancestors for generations to come. Which makes it even more pertinent we work to master these habits. There is so much information out there, and we continue to learn more and more every single day. I encourage you to be a lifelong seeker of knowledge. I truly believe that the day we stop learning is the day that we die. Never stop learning. If you find out information that counters anything in this book, tell me, and we can talk about it. You can reach me at info@coreyhobbs.com. I do not know everything. I will never know everything. I only want to provide information that is going to help people.

Further Readings

I wanted to provide a breakdown of places you can find out more information should you choose to do so. All of these appeared in the reference sections of at least one chapter, so it is likely not the first time you are seeing them.

For more information on food, recipes, and reconstructing your kitchen to suit your needs:

- *Food: What the Heck Should I Eat* - Dr. Mark Hyman
- *Food Fix: How to Save Our Health, Our Economy, Our Communities, and Our Planet -- One Bite at a Time* - Dr. Mark Hyman
- *The Plant Paradox Family Cookbook* - Dr. Steven Gundry
- *Making Healthy Taste Good* - Jason Sani
- *The Grain Brain Cookbook* - Dr. David Perlmutter
- *Good Calories, Bad Calories* - Gary Taubes

For more information on stress, stress management, and sleep:

- *Why Zebras Do Not Get Ulcers* - Dr. Robert Sapolsky
- *Stress Less, Accomplish More: Meditation for Busy Minds* - Emily Fletcher
- *Why We Sleep* - Dr. Matthew Walker

For more information on exercise and performance enhancement:

- *Peak* - Dr. Marc Bubbs
- *Every Day is Game Day* - Mark Verstegen
- *Advances in Functional Training* - Michael Boyle
- *New Functional Training for Sport* - Michael Boyle
- *Poliquin Principles* - Charles Poliquin

For more information on building habits and creating a strong circle of support:

- *Atomic Habits* - James Clear
- *The Culture Code: The Secrets of Highly Successful Groups* - Daniel Coyle
- *Leaders Eat Last* - Simon Sinek

For more on functional medicine:

- *Unconventional Medicine: Join the Revolution to Reinvent Healthcare, Reverse Chronic Disease, and Create a Practice You Love* - Chris Kresser
- *Grain Brain: The Surprising Truth About Wheat, Carbs, and Sugar-Your Brain's Silent Killer* - Dr. David Perlmutter
- *Your Blood Never Lies: How to Read a Blood Test for a Longer, Healthier Life* - Dr. James LaValle

- *Cracking the Metabolic Code: The Nine Keys to Peak Health* - Dr. James LaValle

Free resources to stay on top of new research and information:

- https://www.coreyhobbs.com/blog
- https://blog.designsforhealth.com/
- https://www.thorne.com/take-5-daily
- https://www.livemomentous.com/blogs/momentous
- https://www.precisionnutrition.com/blog
- The Broken Brain Podcast
- The Doctor's Farmacy Podcast
- The Happiness Lab Podcast
- The Genius Life Podcast

Key Takeaways

Finally, if you take away nothing else from this book, I hope that it is the following items. This list of 10 items serves as big picture items to help you have a place to come back to if you need it.

1. Health is the base of all things we do. By prioritizing our health, we can dramatically improve all aspects of our lives.

2. Nobody is perfect. You are going to slip up. That is okay. Do not expect perfection. Forgive yourself and move on to the next opportunity.

3. Every choice we make is an opportunity. Each opportunity can help to get us closer to our goals. Be the person you want to be.

4. Progress is progress. No matter how small the step, a step in the right direction will always get you closer to your goals.

5. We cannot do it alone. Humans are tribal creatures. A large group pulling in the same direction is much more powerful than individuals pulling in many directions

6. Keep it simple. If you are not hungry, do not eat. If you are hungry, eat. When in doubt, eat whole foods that come from quality sources and move often. If this is the only thing we do, we are making tremendous steps towards health.

7.   Track it. If you have a goal, track your progress. It allows you to see how far you have come and how far you might still need to go. You cannot adjust something you are not tracking

8.   Do not forget to live. Dessert every so often is not going to kill you. Enjoy the little moments in life you get with other people. Holidays and vacations are a tremendous opportunity to unwind and strengthen bonds. Do not get so drawn into perfect health that you become a hermit that refuses to do absolutely anything.

9.   Keep learning. New information is coming out all the time. We must be willing to grow. This is especially true if the new information counters what we currently believe. Stay Curious.

10. Experiment. We are not the same. We have different genes, interests, and lifestyles. We need to find what works best in our situation right now, and we should be willing to try something new if the things we are currently trying no longer work in our situation.

All References

Andres, R. H., Ducray, A. D., Schlattner, U., Wallimann, T., & Widmer, H. R. (2008). Functions and effects of creatine in the central nervous system. *Brain Research Bulletin, 76*(4), 329-343.

Asprey, D. (2018). *Game changers: What leaders, innovators, and mavericks do to win at life* HarperCollins.

Asprey, D. (2020). *Superhuman: A bulletproof guide to age backwards and maybe even live forever.* HarperCollins

Bae, J., Park, J., Im, S., & Song, D. (2014). Coffee and health. *Integrative Medicine Research, 3*(4), 189-191.

Brown, B. (2018). *Dare to Lead: Brave Work. Tough Conversations. Whole Hearts*. Random House.

Berardi, J., & Andrews, R. (2010). *The essentials of sport and exercise nutrition*. Precision Nutrition.

Boyle, M. (2004). *Functional training for sports* Human Kinetics Publishers.

Boyle, M. (2016). *New functional training for sports* Human Kinetics.

Bubbs, M. (2019). *Peak: The new science of athletic performance that is revolutionizing sports* Chelsea Green Publishing.

Clear, J. (2018). *Atomic habits: An easy & proven way to build good habits & break bad ones* Avery.

Connolly, F., & White, P. (2017). *Game changer* Simon and Schuster.

Coyle, D. (2018). *The culture code: The secrets of highly successful groups* Bantam.

Craft, L. L., & Perna, F. M. (2004a). The benefits of exercise for the clinically depressed. *Primary Care Companion to the Journal of Clinical Psychiatry, 6*(3), 104.

Craft, L. L., & Perna, F. M. (2004b). The benefits of exercise for the clinically depressed. *Primary Care Companion to the Journal of Clinical Psychiatry, 6*(3), 104.

Crockett, M. J., Clark, L., Lieberman, M. D., Tabibnia, G., & Robbins, T. W. (2010). Impulsive choice and altruistic punishment are correlated and increase in tandem with serotonin depletion. *Emotion, 10*(6), 855.

Davis, D. M., & Hayes, J. A. (2011). What are the benefits of mindfulness? A practice review of psychotherapy-related research. *Psychotherapy, 48*(2), 198.

Dölen, G., Darvishzadeh, A., Huang, K. W., & Malenka, R. C. (2013). Social reward requires coordinated activity of nucleus accumbens oxytocin and serotonin. *Nature, 501*(7466), 179.

Epstein, David. *Range*. Penguin USA, 2020.

Figley, C. R. (2002). Compassion fatigue: Psychotherapists' chronic lack of self-care. *Journal of Clinical Psychology, 58*(11), 1433-1441.

Fletcher, E. (2019). *Stress less, accomplish more: Meditation for busy minds* Boxtree.

Gladwell, V. F., Brown, D. K., Wood, C., Sandercock, G. R., & Barton, J. L. (2013). The great outdoors: How a green exercise environment can benefit all. *Extreme Physiology & Medicine, 2*(1), 3.

Gualano, B., Artioli, G. G., Poortmans, J. R., & Junior, A. H. L. (2010). Exploring the therapeutic role of creatine supplementation. *Amino Acids, 38*(1), 31-44.

Gundry, S. R. (2018). *The plant paradox cookbook: 100 delicious recipes to help you lose weight, heal your gut, and live lectin-free* HarperCollins.

Haff, G. G., & Triplett, N. T. (2015). *Essentials of strength training and conditioning 4th edition* Human kinetics.

Harari, Y. N. (2014). *Sapiens: A brief history of humankind* Random House.

Harari, Y. N. (2016). *Homo deus: A brief history of tomorrow* Random House.

Hoenselaar, R. (2012). Saturated fat and cardiovascular disease: The discrepancy between the scientific literature and dietary advice. *Nutrition, 28*(2), 118-123.

Horowitz, S. (2010). Health benefits of meditation: What the newest research shows. *Alternative and Complementary Therapies, 16*(4), 223-228.

https://www.precisionnutrition.com/diets-are-dead

http://main.poliquingroup.com/ArticlesMultimedia/Articles/Article/2793/Seven_Reasons_To_Never_Diet.aspx

https://blog.designsforhealth.com/teenagers-insufficient-sleep-obesity-gotosleep

https://blog.designsforhealth.com/Insulin%20Sensitivity%20and%20Sleep%2C%20or%20Lack%20Thereof

https://blog.bulletproof.com/how-to-hack-your-sleep the-art-and-science-of-sleeping

https://www.kissthegroundmovie.com

https://www.precisionnutrition.com/calorie-control-guide-infographic

https://www.instagram.com/p/B6fmAOyJWYq/

https://www.thepowerofwhenquiz.com

https://www.headspace.com/science/meditation-benefits

https://www.tenpercent.com/

Hyman, M. (2018). *Food: What the heck should I eat?* Hachette UK.

Hyman, M. (2020). *Food Fix: How to Save Our Health, Our Economy, Our Communities, and Our Planet -- One Bite at a Time.* Little, Brown Spark

Jones, D. S., Bland, J. S., & Quinn, S. (2005). What is functional medicine. *Textbook of Functional Medicine,* 5-14.

Klok, M. D., Jakobsdottir, S., & Drent, M. L. (2007). The role of leptin and ghrelin in the regulation of food intake and body weight in humans: A review. *Obesity Reviews, 8*(1), 21-34.

Kresser, C. (2017). *Unconventional medicine: Join the revolution to reinvent healthcare, reverse chronic disease, and create a practice you love* Lioncrest Publishing.

Kumar, S. (2016). Burnout and doctors: Prevalence, prevention and intervention. Paper presented at the *Healthcare, 4*(3) 37.

LaValle, J. B. (2013). *Your blood never lies: How to read a blood test for a longer, healthier life* Square One Publishers, Inc.

LaValle, J. B., & Yale, S. L. (2004). *Cracking the metabolic code: The nine keys to peak health* Basic Health Publications, Inc.

Learney, P. (2014). *N1 nutritional programming: The fundamentals of nutritional programming.* ACA.

Levine, J. A. (2002). Non-exercise activity thermogenesis (NEAT). *Best Practice & Research Clinical Endocrinology & Metabolism, 16*(4), 679-702.

Luna, R. A., & Foster, J. A. (2015). Gut brain axis: Diet microbiota interactions and implications for modulation of anxiety and depression. *Current Opinion in Biotechnology, 32,* 35-41.

Lunenburg, F. C. (2011). Goal-setting theory of motivation. *International Journal of Management, Business, and Administration, 15*(1), 1-6.

Lynch, B. (2018). *Dirty genes* Harper One, New York.

Malhotra, A., Redberg, R. F., & Meier, P. (2017). Saturated fat does not clog the arteries: Coronary heart disease is a chronic inflammatory condition, the risk of which can be effectively reduced from healthy lifestyle interventions. *BMJ Publishing Group Ltd and British Association of Sport and Exercise Medicine,*

Medina, J. (2011). *Brain rules: 12 principles for surviving and thriving at work, home, and school* ReadHowYouWant. com.

Neth, B. J., & Craft, S. (2017). Insulin resistance and alzheimer's disease: Bioenergetic linkages. *Frontiers in Aging Neuroscience, 9,* 345.

Perlmutter, D. (2014). *The grain brain cookbook* Little Brown & Company.

Perlmutter, D. (2018). *Grain brain: The surprising truth about wheat, carbs, and sugar--your brain's silent killers* Hachette UK.

Pollack, G. H. (2013a). The fourth phase of water. *Ebner & Sons Publishers, Seattle, Washington,*

Pollack, G. H. (2013b). The fourth phase of water: Beyond solid. *Liquid, and Vapor,*

Poliquin, Charles. Poliquin Principles: Successful Methods for Strength and Mass Development. Poliquin Performance Centers, 2006.

Rose, T. (2016). *The end of average: How to succeed in a world that values sameness* Penguin UK.

Ross, R. G., Hunter, S. K., Hoffman, M. C., McCarthy, L., Chambers, B. M., Law, A. J., Freedman, R. (2015). Perinatal phosphatidylcholine supplementation and early childhood behavior problems: Evidence for CHRNA7 moderation. *American Journal of Psychiatry, 173*(5), 509-516.

Rowan, A. E., Kueffner, T. E., & Stavrianeas, S. (2012). Short duration high-intensity interval training improves aerobic conditioning of female college soccer players. *International Journal of Exercise Science, 5*(3), 6.

Sakellaris, G., Kotsiou, M., Tamiolaki, M., Kalostos, G., Tsapaki, E., Spanaki, M., Evangeliou, A. (2006). Prevention of complications related to traumatic brain injury in children and adolescents with creatine administration: An open label randomized pilot study. *Journal of Trauma and Acute Care Surgery, 61*(2), 322-329.

Sapolsky, R. M. (2017). *Behave: The biology of humans at our best and worst* Penguin.

Sapolsky, R. M. (2004). *Why zebras do not get ulcers: The acclaimed guide to stress, stress-related diseases, and coping-now revised and updated* Holt paperbacks.

Saslow, L. R., Summers, C., Aikens, J. E., & Unwin, D. J. (2018). Outcomes of a digitally delivered low-carbohydrate type 2 diabetes self-management program: 1-year results of a single-arm longitudinal study. *JMIR Diabetes, 3*(3), e12.

Scheier, M. F., & Carver, C. S. (1993). On the power of positive thinking: The benefits of being optimistic. *Current Directions in Psychological Science, 2*(1), 26-30.

Schjerve, I. E., Tyldum, G. A., Tjønna, A. E., Stølen, T., Loennechen, J. P., Hansen, H. E., Najjar, S. M. (2008). Both aerobic endurance and strength training programmes improve cardiovascular health in obese adults. *Clinical Science, 115*(9), 283-293.

Schreiner, I., & Malcolm, J. P. (2008). The benefits of mindfulness meditation: Changes in emotional states of depression, anxiety, and stress. *Behaviour Change, 25*(3), 156-168.

Shanahan, C. (2017). *Deep nutrition: Why your genes need traditional food.* Flatiron Books.

Shonin, E., Van Gordon, W., & Griffiths, M. D. (2013). Meditation as medication: Are attitudes changing? *Br J Gen Pract, 63*(617), 654.

Sinek, S. (2009). *Start with why: How great leaders inspire everyone to take action* Penguin.

Sinek, S. (2014). *Leaders eat last: Why some teams pull together and others do not* Penguin.

Suez, J., Korem, T., Zeevi, D., Zilberman-Schapira, G., Thaiss, C. A., Maza, O., Weinberger, A. (2014). Artificial sweeteners induce glucose intolerance by altering the gut microbiota. *Nature, 514*(7521), 181.

Sullivan, P. G., Geiger, J. D., Mattson, M. P., & Scheff, S. W. (2000). Dietary supplement creatine protects against traumatic brain injury. *Annals of Neurology, 48*(5), 723-729.

Swithers, S. E. (2013). Artificial sweeteners produce the counterintuitive effect of inducing metabolic derangements. *Trends in Endocrinology & Metabolism, 24*(9), 431-441.

Taheri, S., Lin, L., Austin, D., Young, T., & Mignot, E. (2004). Short sleep duration is associated with reduced leptin, elevated ghrelin, and increased body mass index. *PLoS Medicine, 1*(3), e62.

Taleb, N. N. (2012). *Antifragile: How to live in a world we do not understand* Allen Lane London.

Taleb, N. N. (2020). *Skin in the game: Hidden asymmetries in daily life* Random House Trade Paperbacks.

Tarnopolsky, M. A., & Beal, M. F. (2001). Potential for creatine and other therapies targeting cellular energy dysfunction in neurological disorders. *Annals of Neurology, 49*(5), 561-574.

Taubes, G. (2007). *Good calories, bad calories* Anchor.

Tsutsumi, T., Don, B. M., Zaichkowsky, L. D., & Delizonna, L. L. (1997a). Physical fitness and psychological benefits of strength training in community dwelling older adults. *Applied Human Science, 16*(6), 257-266.

Tsutsumi, T., Don, B. M., Zaichkowsky, L. D., & Delizonna, L. L. (1997b). Physical fitness and psychological benefits of strength training in community dwelling older adults. *Applied Human Science, 16*(6), 257-266.

Verstegen, M., & Williams, P. (2014). *Every day is game day: Train like the pros with a no-holds-barred exercise and nutrition plan for peak performance* Penguin.

Vitaliano, P. P., Scanlan, J. M., Zhang, J., Savage, M. V., Hirsch, I. B., & Siegler, I. C. (2002). A path model of chronic stress, the metabolic syndrome, and coronary heart disease. *Psychosomatic Medicine, 64*(3), 418-435.

Walker, M. (2017). *Why we sleep: Unlocking the power of sleep and dreams* Simon and Schuster.

Zaidi, F. B. A. (2019). Organizational role stress and job burnout among doctors. *Omegademy Journal of Psychological Research, 1*(1), 13-26.

About the Author

Corey Hobbs

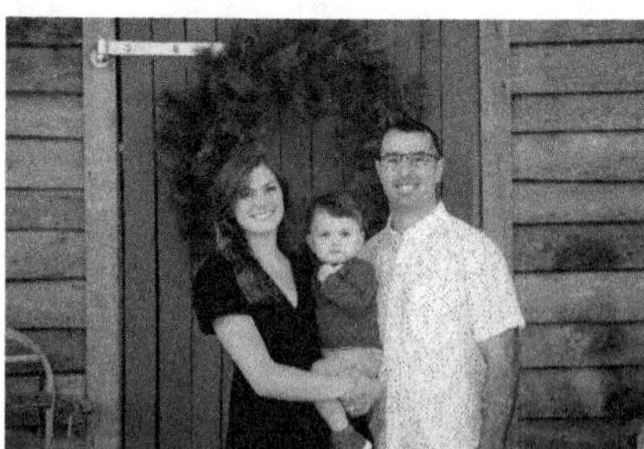

Corey and his family currently reside in Nashville, Tennessee. Corey Attended the United States Military Academy where he played football and majored in Kinesiology. Following his time in the Army, Corey began his career as a Strength and Conditioning Coach at Tennessee Technology University where he oversaw the Strength and Conditioning programs for Women's Soccer, Women's Golf, Men's Golf, and Co-Ed Cheer teams. He also assisted with the Football program. He decided to leave TTU to be closer to home and maximize the time he has with his family. He continues coaching and working with athletes of various levels creating unique strength and conditioning programs paired with nutritional education based on their unique needs to maximize the Four Pillars of Health. As of publishing, Corey is working towards his Master's in Nutrition in order to become a Registered Dietitian. He plans on integrating Functional Medicine principles into his practice as a Strength and Conditioning Coach and dietitian.